NEUROLOGY – LABORATORY AND
CLINICAL RESEARCH DEVELOPMENTS

NEUROLOGICAL DISEASES

FROM DIAGNOSIS TO TREATMENT

NEUROLOGY – LABORATORY AND CLINICAL RESEARCH DEVELOPMENTS

Additional books and e-books in this series can be found on Nova's website under the Series tab.

NEUROLOGY – LABORATORY AND
CLINICAL RESEARCH DEVELOPMENTS

NEUROLOGICAL DISEASES FROM DIAGNOSIS TO TREATMENT

PHILIP L. THYGESEN
EDITOR

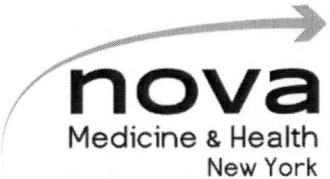

Copyright © 2019 by Nova Science Publishers, Inc.

All rights reserved. No part of this book may be reproduced, stored in a retrieval system or transmitted in any form or by any means: electronic, electrostatic, magnetic, tape, mechanical photocopying, recording or otherwise without the written permission of the Publisher.

We have partnered with Copyright Clearance Center to make it easy for you to obtain permissions to reuse content from this publication. Simply navigate to this publication's page on Nova's website and locate the "Get Permission" button below the title description. This button is linked directly to the title's permission page on copyright.com. Alternatively, you can visit copyright.com and search by title, ISBN, or ISSN.

For further questions about using the service on copyright.com, please contact:
Copyright Clearance Center
Phone: +1-(978) 750-8400   Fax: +1-(978) 750-4470   E-mail: info@copyright.com

NOTICE TO THE READER

The Publisher has taken reasonable care in the preparation of this book, but makes no expressed or implied warranty of any kind and assumes no responsibility for any errors or omissions. No liability is assumed for incidental or consequential damages in connection with or arising out of information contained in this book. The Publisher shall not be liable for any special, consequential, or exemplary damages resulting, in whole or in part, from the readers' use of, or reliance upon, this material. Any parts of this book based on government reports are so indicated and copyright is claimed for those parts to the extent applicable to compilations of such works.

Independent verification should be sought for any data, advice or recommendations contained in this book. In addition, no responsibility is assumed by the Publisher for any injury and/or damage to persons or property arising from any methods, products, instructions, ideas or otherwise contained in this publication.

This publication is designed to provide accurate and authoritative information with regard to the subject matter covered herein. It is sold with the clear understanding that the Publisher is not engaged in rendering legal or any other professional services. If legal or any other expert assistance is required, the services of a competent person should be sought. FROM A DECLARATION OF PARTICIPANTS JOINTLY ADOPTED BY A COMMITTEE OF THE AMERICAN BAR ASSOCIATION AND A COMMITTEE OF PUBLISHERS.

Additional color graphics may be available in the e-book version of this book.

Library of Congress Cataloging-in-Publication Data

ISBN: 978-1-53616-205-9
Library of Congress Control Number:2019948966

Published by Nova Science Publishers, Inc. † New York

CONTENTS

Preface		vii
Chapter 1	Therapeutic Apheresis in Neurologic Diseases with Immunological Origin *Rolf Bambauer and Ralf Schiel*	1
Chapter 2	Possible Therapeutic Effects of Ceftriaxone in Aluminum Neurotoxicity When Applied before and after Aluminum *Ankica Jelenković, Marina D. Jovanović, Ivana Stevanović and Vera Prokić*	27
Chapter 3	Implementation of a Concept of Neuropalliative and Rehabilitation Care for Patients with Progressive, Neurological Disease in the Czech Republic: A Qualitative Study *Radka Bužgová, Radka Kozáková and Michal Bar*	73
Index		97
Related Nova Publications		101

PREFACE

In Neurological Diseases: From Diagnosis to Treatment, the authors provide an overview of the most important pathogenic aspects which indicate that therapeutic apheresis can be a supportive therapy in systemic autoimmune diseases such as renal and neurological disorders.

Next, the authors examine whether ceftriaxone could influence aluminum brain neurotoxic effects through a study wherein four groups of adult male Wistar rats underwent four different treatments via stereotaxic brain surgery.

The concluding study proposes an implementation of a concept of neuropalliative and rehabilitative care for patients with progressive neurological disease within the systems of health and social care in the Czech Republic.

Chapter 1 - Since the mid 1970s, membrane modules became available, and the plasma separation techniques have gained in importance in the past few years. The advantages of this method are a complete separation of the corpuscular components from the plasma and due to increased blood flow rate higher efficacy. Systemic autoimmune diseases based on an immune pathogenesis produce autoantibodies and circulating immune complexes, which cause inflammation in the tissues of various organs. In most cases, these diseases have a bad prognosis without treatment. Therapeutic apheresis (TA) in combination with immunosuppressive therapies has led to a steady increase in survival rates over the last 45 years. The updated information on immunology and molecular biology of different immunologic diseases are discussed in relation to the rationale for therapeutic apheresis therapy and its place in combination with other modern treatments. The different diseases can treated by various apheresis methods such as therapeutic plasma exchange (TPE) with substitution solution, or with online plasma or blood purification using adsorption columns which contain biological or non biological agents. Here the authors provide an overview of the most important pathogenic aspects indicating that TA can be a supportive therapy in systemic autoimmune diseases such as renal and neurological disorders. For the immunological diseases that can treated with TA, the guidelines of the Apheresis Application Committee of the American Society for Apheresis are cited.

Chapter 2 - Ceftriaxone, a β-lactam antibiotic primarily applied for its antimicrobial effects, in the last decade was suggested to be neuroprotective as well due to its abilities to increase the expression of membrane-bound glutamate transporter EAAT2/GLT-1 and counteract glutamate-mediated neurotoxicity. The dysfunction of GLT-1 transporter and the consequent accumulation of excessive extracellular glutamate is correlated with multiple neurodegenerative pathologies. Oxidative stress, one of the multifold and complex variables responsible for the development of these diseases, is also recognized in aluminum neurotoxicity. Furthermore, aluminum has almost unambiguously been shown to take part in the etiopathogenetic processes of Alzheimer's and other neurodegenerative diseases. Due to all the previously mentioned facts, it was of interest to examine whether ceftriaxone could influence the aluminum brain neurotoxic effects. To do so, the authors subjected four groups of adult male Wistar rats to four different treatments *via* stereotaxic brain surgery. Saline and aluminum chloride (3.7×10^{-4}g/kg) were applied intrahippocampally. Aluminum was given prior to, as well as after five consecutive days of ceftriaxone treatment (200mg/kg body weight, applied intraperitoneally). Rats were decapitated on the 13th day of recovery after surgery. In the four brain regions (forebrain cortex, striatum, basal forebrain and hippocampus) the activity of cytochrome c oxidase and glucose-6-phosphate dehydrogenase were determined, as well as the level of reduced glutathione. Based on the obtained results, it was evident that ceftriaxone significantly attenuated the detrimental effects of aluminum on all of the analyzed brain parameters, but also it restored them entirely. Besides, ceftriaxone pre-treatment displayed stronger effects than the after-treatment. Accordingly, the ability of ceftriaxone to alleviate the harmful protoxidative effects of aluminum in the brain can be a new approach to combating oxidative stress that is involved in the pathogenesis of various brain disorders.

Chapter 3 - Palliative care provided to patients with progressive neurological disease (PND) can result in an improvement of the quality of their life. The aim of the qualitative research was to propose an implementation of a concept of neuropalliative and rehabilitation care for patients with PND within the system of health- and social care in the Czech Republic. The research included focus groups (n = 4) comprising 33 participants. The method of thematic analysis was used to analyze the obtained data. The research included 33 participants - 30 professionals working with PND patients, 2 hospital chaplains, and a patient with PD. A three-level model was suggested consisting of the following phases: 1/ supportive care / rehabilitation, 2/ neuropalliative rehabilitation, 3/ specialist palliative care. Efficient communication methods, support of the family, and identification of suitable patients were emphasized in the individual phases of provided care. For further research, the authors recommend verifying the efficiency of the three-level concept of the neuropalliative and rehabilitation care in an intervention study.

In: Neurological Diseases
Editor: Philip L. Thygesen

ISBN: 978-1-53616-205-9
© 2019 Nova Science Publishers, Inc.

Chapter 1

THERAPEUTIC APHERESIS IN NEUROLOGIC DISEASES WITH IMMUNOLOGICAL ORIGIN

Rolf Bambauer[1,*] *and Ralf Schiel*[2]
[1]Formerly: Institute for Blood Purification,
Homburg, Germany
[2]Inselklinik Heringsdorf GmbH, Seeheilbad
Heringsdorf, Germany

ABSTRACT

Since the mid 1970s, membrane modules became available, and the plasma separation techniques have gained in importance in the past few years. The advantages of this method are a complete separation of the corpuscular components from the plasma and due to increased blood flow rate higher efficacy. Systemic autoimmune diseases based on an immune pathogenesis produce autoantibodies and circulating immune complexes, which cause inflammation in the tissues of various organs. In most cases, these diseases have a bad prognosis without treatment. Therapeutic apheresis (TA) in combination with immunosuppressive therapies has led to a steady increase in survival rates over the last 45 years. The updated

---

[*] Corresponding Author's Email: rolf.bambauer@t-online.de.

information on immunology and molecular biology of different immunologic diseases are discussed in relation to the rationale for therapeutic apheresis therapy and its place in combination with other modern treatments. The different diseases can treated by various apheresis methods such as therapeutic plasma exchange (TPE) with substitution solution, or with online plasma or blood purification using adsorption columns which contain biological or non biological agents. Here the authors provide an overview of the most important pathogenic aspects indicating that TA can be a supportive therapy in systemic autoimmune diseases such as renal and neurological disorders. For the immunological diseases that can treated with TA, the guidelines of the Apheresis Application Committee of the American Society for Apheresis are cited.

Keywords: therapeutic apheresis, immunologic diseases, therapeutic plasma exchange, immunoadsorption, neurologic diseases, immunological disorders

INTRODUCTION

"The ancient medical belief that removal of a patient's blood can also lead to the removal of his disease" would not withstand a critical examination by modern medicine, but now the basic principle put on a rational basis, is returning to practised medicine [1]. Up to now TA has proved itself in a series of immunological, metabolic diseases, and intoxications. With more selective plasma separation and immunoadsorption (IA) with immobilized monoclonal or polyclonal antibodies etc. have secured their place in clinical routine, one will have taken a great step nearer to the wish of our medical ancestors of removing "the disease factors from the blood" and will able to provide improved treatment for many diseases [1].

The introduction of hollow fiber modules in TA brings a complete separation of the corpuscular components from the plasma and due to increased blood flow rate higher efficacy [1]. TA using centrifuges has shorter treatment times such as TA using hollow fibers shown by Hafer et al. is no advantage [2]. More important is to keep the blood levels with antibodies, and/or pathogenic substances on a very low level over longer time during the treatment. In this situation the substances which should eliminated could invade into the intravascular space and eliminated by the membrane separators.

The conventional TPE equipments are, however, not perfect, because the filtered plasma fractions have to discard. Substitution solutions supplemented with human albumin, plasma substitutes (e.g., gelatine solutions), or fresh frozen plasma are used to replace the discarded fractions [1]. Since several years plasma perfusion methods such as IA or other selective plasma adsorption methods are available without the use of a substitution solution.

The cause of autoimmune reactions is still generally unknown. The spectrum of autoimmune diseases ranges from those diseases in which autoimmunization are solely responsible for the disease condition (e.g., autoimmune hemolytic anemia), to those in which it possibly has a major influence on the further course of the disease (e.g., rheumatoid arthritis), and those in which the autoimmunization phenomena are probably only of diagnostic importance [1]. The autoantibodies (auto-abs), which activate immunological processes that are self-destructive for the organism, have their effects in different ways. These autoantibodies can also directed at all blood cells.

In nearly all immune response adhesions of leucocytes to other cell to other types and between different types of leucocytes are involved. Leucocytes have to attach to stromal cells in the bone marrow and in the thymus to receive proper differentiation signals. Later they must attach to endothelial cells as they leave the blood circulation and enter tissues, where they adhere to macromolecules of the extracellular matrix. All intercellular interactions are mediated by various pairs of adhesion molecules [3].

Inflammation is a complex set of events accompanied by the release of many different soluble substances such as antibodies that diffuse away from the side of their production. Autoantibodies can detected in all tissues and can directed against many non-hematogenous tissues. Antibodies of the IgG class can transverse blood vessel wall and enter extravascular tissue spaces. Antibodies of the IgM and also IgA and IgD class usually cannot cross blood vessel walls [1, 4]. Autoantibodies are not necessarily primarily autoaggressive or destructive. They only lead to inflammatory tissue reaction when, through their binding to cells and through complement activation, the reaction chain of the serum complement system is triggered [1]. Circulating antibodies bind the offending antigens and participate in several other functions. Together they can trigger tissue inflammation ranging from slight vascular irritation to necrosis. The serum concentration of the individual components varies considerably, so that here the concept of the "limiting factor" applies.

Autoantibodies can, however, have a serious effect on a given organ even without the activation of the complement system, namely when either functionally important receptors are blocked by antibodies or else important proteins are rendered inactive through the union with antibodies, such as hormones or enzymes. Myasthenia gravis is a classic example for a receptor blockade [5]. These principles of receptor blockade are used since several years in medicaments for example as angiotensin converting enzyme inhibitors (ACE) or angiotensin II type receptor blockers [1]. Autoantibodies can also block the physiological decomposition of enzymes which results in an extreme disorder of the regulatory mechanisms.

Immune complex (IC) is a physiological process and serves to eliminate foreign material, such as bacteria, their components and viruses. If such ICs are formed, they are removed from the blood by the adhesion of the Fc-fragments of the antibodies to the corresponding phagocyte receptors in the liver and spleen. Phagocytosis can even enhance if the ICs activate the complement system (immune clearance). However, if not all the ICs are eliminated quickly enough in this way, then they can establish themselves in the intima of the vessels and from there trigger inflammatory lesions through local activation of the complement system [1]. The ICs probably first form in situ; the antigen adheres to the basal membrane and binds circulating antibodies. If this is correct, then IC deposition processes in tissue are not necessarily detectable through serum IC determination, as, on the other hand, circulating ICs (CIC) must do not indicate organ damage.

Immune complexes deposit preferentially in certain sites throughout the body, the kidneys, the joints, the lungs and the skin. The kidney accumulates IC because the blood pressure in the glomerular capillaries is four times higher than in other capillaries and because the glomerulus retains immune ICs by a simple filtering effect. Similarly, ICs may also accumulate on other body filters; the ciliary body eye, where aqueous humor forms, and the choroid plexus in the brain, where cerebrospinal fluid is produced.

Circulating immune complexes are involved in the regulation of various immune phenomena. These ICs interacts with the Fc and/or antigen receptors of the T, B, NK cells and macrophages. They correlate to the primary and secondary immune response [6]. The elimination of the CICs plays an important therapeutic role. It is possible to interrupt the pathological process by eliminating antibodies by TA. The methods of TA such as TPE, double filtration plasma exchange (DFPP) or the different semiselective or selective plasma exchange methods available are published elsewhere and discussed in detail by Bambauer et al. [1, 7, 8].

Therapeutic Apheresis

TPE was explored in the treatment of a variety of autoimmune syndromes. There are only a few prospective controlled trials available that are of adequate statistical power to allow definitive conclusions to reach regarding the therapeutic value of TA. This drawback reflects, in part, the relative rarity of most of the disorders under investigation. To compensate, many investigators have understandably grouped heterogenous diseases together, often retrospectively, and used historical controls. The latter design is potentially hazardous, given that earlier diagnosis, recognition of milder cases, and improved general care over time may be lost as a benefit of TPE.

For those diseases for which the use of TA is discussed, the guidelines on the use of TA from the Apheresis Applications Committee (AAC) of the American Society for Apheresis (ASFA) are cited [9, 10]. Since the introduction of hollow fiber modules in TPE, this therapy method is mostly used in nephrology, as many of these membranes can be used with the currently available dialysis equipment.

Therapeutic Plasma exchange uses membranes for plasma filtration separation and fractionation may be distinguished from conventional dialysis membranes and high-flux membranes used in hemofiltration by their very high or select passage of plasma proteins. The advantages of membrane plasmapheresis include its simplicity to use with blood pumps and no observed white blood cell or platelet loss, compared with centrifuges. The permeability of all these membranes for macromolecular substances reaches a molecular mass of 0.2×10^6 to 0.5×10^6 Dalton. The limit of permeability can be reduced by means of changes in the spin process [1].

Cascade Filtration (CF), membrane differential filtration (MDF) seems to be superior to conventional plasmapheresis but less effective than adsorption or precipitation techniques [1, 11, 12]. The CF was developed by Agishi et al. 1980 in Japan and was the first semiselective technique. [11]. Secondary membrane in cascade filtration has a cut off of approximately one million daltons. LDL particles with a molecular weight of approximately 2,300,000 daltons are thus retained by this membrane. All other molecules, which are larger than one million daltons are also retained, while plasma components smaller than one million daltons pass through the membrane and are returned to the patient. With a treatment of 1.0 – 1.2 total plasma volume (TPV), antibodies can be reduced by approximately 35–50 percent of the original value [12]. Due to irregular pore distribution with different diameters in the secondary membrane, plasma components with smaller molecular weight can also retained, such as fibrinogen (MW: Å 340,000), HDL (MW: Å 400,000), and IgM (MW: Å 1,000,000) [13]. To reduce fibrinogen, MDF is an effective method. With synthetic secondary membranes and newer types of machines, better effectiveness and selectivity in the separation of the blood components can reach. MDF is as safe and effective. Fully automated apheresis machines have been developed so that continuous manual steering of flows and blood pressures is no longer required (Octo Nova/Diamed, Germany) [13].

Immunoadsorption (IA) was first described by Stoffel et al. in 1981 as LDL-apheresis through sepharose columns coated with LDL antibodies, or other antibodies [14]. The autoantibodies in the plasma after primary separation are adsorbed in the columns onto the antibodies. This is a reversible antigen-antibody bond accord based on the principle of affinity chromatography. The 2 columns contain 300–320 ml or less volume of sepharose particles. Before one column is saturated with the absorbed autoantibodies (600–800 mL plasma), the plasma flow is switched to the other column; while one column is used for adsorption, the off-line column is regenerated with neutral saline buffer solution, lysine buffer (pH 2.4), and neutral buffer again. The treated plasma is then mixed with the cellular components of the blood and returned to the patient. The whole procedure takes 2.5–3 hours with the computerized apheresis monitor [1]. After the treatment, the columns are rinsed, and filled with sterile solution.

Required volume of plasma of 3 – 10 L can be perfused in one treatment session. The advantage of this method is the high selectivity, effectiveness for all apo-B-containing lipoproteins, and regenerating capacity of the columns. The disadvantage is the high expenditure required not only for the treatment itself, but also for the regeneration process [14]. A long-term basis that is to say, at least 20 times per patient is only viable for the high costs of the columns. At a perfusion of 1.2- 2.4 TPV per session, the autoantibodies are reduced to 30–40 percent of the original concentration. HDL, serum proteins, immunoglobulins, and fibrinogen, and others drop by approximately 15–20 percent and return to their normal level, after approximately 24 hours. The system is safe and effective in clinical use, even in long term treatment [14].

The other therapeutic apheresis methods such as the Heparin-induced LDL precipitation (HELP), LDL-adsorption (dextran sulfate, Liposorber) and the LDL hemoperfusion DALI and Liposorber D systems are not used in neurologic diseases.

Neurologic Disorders

Neurologic disorders constitute the largest group of indications for TA [15]. Severe central nervous system (CNS) involvement is associated with poor prognosis, and high mortality rate. High dose steroid and cyclophosphamide (oral or intravenous) are the first choice of drugs in the treatment; TA, intravenous immune globuline (IVIG), thalidomide, intratechal treatment may be valuable in treatment resistant, and serious cases. Table 1 shows the most of the neurological diseases that have treated with TPE with the categories and the recommendation grade (RG) of the guidelines from the AAC of the ASFA [9, 10].

Acute Inflammatory Demyelinating Polyneuropathy (AIDP, Guillain-Barré Syndrome, GBS)

AIPD is an autoaggressive disorder that develops subsequent to infectious diseases and as a result of other noxae [1]. It is an acute polyradiculitis, which mostly affects the distal and proximal muscles of the extremities, as well as the trunk muscles and can progress with severe ascending paralysis, ending in respiratory paralysis [16]. The clinical symptomatology is a progressive weakness of acute onset of members, usually distal and symmetrical, with hyporeflexia or areflexia. The progression is rapid with possible involvement of cranial nerves, weakness of the diaphragmatic muscle [17]. Most patients with AIDP have inflammatory, predominantly demyelinating polyneuropathy [1]. This acute progressive disease, leading to rising paralysis, usually reaches its height within one to two weeks; 25 percent of all patients require artificial ventilation. AIDP occurs in one out of 50,000 persons each year in the industrial nations, regardless of gender or age.

The pathophysiologic mechanism has not been established completely, but in many cases, an antecedent infection by campylobacter jejuni leads to the production of antibodies directed against certain epitopes of the bacterium that also destroy the myelin sheath of the peripheral nerve. This phenomenon has been described as molecular mimicry [18]. The spectrum of organisms responsible for infections can trigger GBS ranges from Epstein-Barr virus to mycoplasma, herpes zoster, and mumps virus, borrelia to the HIV viruses. The autoaggressive disease is an acute polyradiculitis, often an inflammatory demyelinating polyradiculitis [1]. In recent years, the triggering causes have described as being:

1) Antibodies against peripheral nerves, in particular against myelin;
2) Circulating immune complexes;
3) Complement activation in the cerebrospinal fluid and in serum;
4) Other inflammatory mediators and cytokines; and
5) A disorder in cell-related immunity [1].

Spontaneous recovery normally occurs between the 2nd and 4th week of illness, and, in 75 percent of the patients, it can even occur after several months of illness. Due to remaining damage and relapses, lethality is between 5 and 25 percent after one year [1]. The rationale for TA is based on the humeral and cellular immune dysfunction in this disease. In his reports Weinstein discussed this rationale well and described a large number of immunological features [19, 20].

IVIG has also been shown to be effective in the treatment of AIDP. In a recent large international randomized study of TPE, IVIG, and combined treatments in AIDP, all three modalities were effective [17, 21, 22]. While no significant statistical differences were noted between the groups, TPE was noted to be better than IVIG, and the combination was better than either of the treatments alone and this combination is recommended as the first-line therapy [22 – 24].

In recent years, researchers have applied a combination therapy of TPE or IA following by IgG (0.4g/kg BW for 5 days) [1]. Haupt et al. reported results which suggesting that such a combination treatment of AIDP may be superior to plasma exchange alone [25]. Accordingly, with TPE treatment in GBS, it was possible to reduce the costs by between 30 to 40 percent in America, due to the shorter periods of inpatient treatment and shorter duration of artificial respiration [1]. Lin et al. reported in 2015 of 60 patients with GBS treated with DFPP. They found a complication rate of 18.3% [26]. Besides adult patients, children seem to benefit from apheresis therapy in steroid resistant inflammatory demyelinating conditions [27].

In the guidelines on the use of TA in clinical practice-evidence-based approach from the AAC of the ASFA, the AIDP has the category I with the RG 1A (Table 1) [9, 10]. Category I means TPE and IA are effective in 55 - 100% and both are accepted as first-line therapy [28]. The main etiology of

AIDP is autoimmune antibody-mediated damage to the peripheral nerve myelin [9]. Several controlled trials comparing TPE to supportive care alone indicate TPE treatment can accelerate motor recovery, decrease time on the ventilator, and speed attainment of other clinical milestones. While recovery with TPE is improved, the duration of disability from AIDP remains significant. The Cochrane Neuromuscular Disease Group review of TPE in AIDP found that TPE is most effective when initiated within 7 days of disease onset [10].

Chronic Inflammatory Demyelinating Polyradiculoneuropathy (CIPD)

CIPD is a rare uncommon progressive or relapsing paralysing disease caused by inflammation of the peripheral nerves [10]. Neurologic symptoms are decreased sensation, diminished or absent reflexes, elevated cerebrospinal fluid level, and evidence of demyelination. The acquired disorder of the peripheral nervous system (CIPD) has probably an auto-immune pathogenesis. But a single autoantibody has not found to act as a biomarker for CIPD overall, specific autoantibodies have identified in the peripheral nerves of about 10% of the patients [29]. The nature of the responsible auto-antigens is unclear in most patients. The frequency of such antibodies is significantly greater in CIPD patients than in normal control subjects [30].

Recent clinical trials have confirmed the short term efficacy of IVIG, prednisone and TPE. In the absence of better evidence about long-term efficacy, corticosteroids or IVIG are usually favored because of convenience. Benefit following introduction of azathioprine, cyclophosphamide, cyclosporin, other immunosuppressive agents, and interferon-β and $-\alpha$ has reported but randomized trials are needed to confirm these benefits [29, 31]. Therefore Hughes et al. recommended in 2006 that the principle treatments are:

Table 1. TA in neurologic diseases with immunologic origin

(Category I: accepted for TA as first-line therapy; Category II: accepted for TA as second-line therapy; Category III: not accepted for TA, decision should be individualized; Category IV: not accepted for TA, approval is desirable if TA is undertaken [9, 10])

	Apheresis Applications Committee of the ASFA, 2013, 2016 [9, 10]					
	TA modality	Category	Recommendation grade	Treated volume (TPV)	Replacement solution	Frequency
Acute inflammatory demyelinating Polyneuropathy (AIDP)	TPE,	I	1A			
Chronic inflammatory demyelinating polyradiculoneuropathy (CIPD)	IA-Protein-A	I	1B	1-1.5		
Myasthenia gravis (MG) (moderate, severe)	TPE	I	1A	1-1.5	human-albumin-electrolyte solution	daily or every other day
Pre-thymectomy		I	1C			
Multiple sclerosis (MS)	TPE			1-1.5		
- acute MS		II	1B			
-chronic progressive		III	2B			

Table 1. (Continued)

	Apheresis Applications Committee of the ASFA, 2013, 2016 [9, 10]					
	TA modality	Category	Recommendation grade	Treated volume (TPV)	Replacement solution	Frequency
Pediatric autoimmune neuropsychiatric Disorder associated with streptococcal Infections (PANDAS), Sydenham's chorea	TPE	I I	1B 1B	1-1.5	human-albumin-electrolyte solution	daily or every other day, 14 days
Chronic focal encephalitis (CFE) (Rasmussen encephalitis)	TPE, IA	III III	2C 2 C	1-1.5		daily or every other day
Acute disseminated encephalitis (ADEM)	TPE	II	2C	1-1.5		
Lambert-Eaton myasthenic syndrome	TPE	II	2C	1-1.5		
Miller-Fisher syndrome (MFS)	TPE	III	2C	1-1.5		

IA-Protein-A: Immunoadsorption on protein-A (Immunosorba®, Prosorba®, Fresenius, Germany).

- intravenous immunoglobulin or corticosteroids should be considered in sensory and motor CIPD,
- IVIG should be considered as the initial treatment in pure motor CIPD,
- if IVIG and corticosteroids are ineffective TA should be considered,
- if the response is inadequate or the maintenance doses of the initial treatment are high,
- combination treatments or adding an immunosuppressant or immunomodulatory drugs could be considered,
- symptomatic treatment and multidisciplinary management should be considered [31].

IVIG, corticosteroids, and TPE or IA are the first-line therapies for the treatment of CIPD [32]. In the guidelines of the AAC of the ASFA, the CIPD has the category I and the RG 1B (Table 1) [9, 10]. TPE or IA are indicated when patients do not respond to corticosteroids and/or IVIG treatment. If a rapid response is needed, than TPE or IA are indicated [33].

Myasthenia Gravis (MG)

MG is a disease caused by autoantibodies, which are directed against acetylcholine receptors of the skeletal muscles. The acetylcholine receptor antibodies (Ach-R-ab) belong to a heterogenous group of polyclonal abs, which are directed against various sections of the post-synaptic receptor molecule. Due to blockage of the receptors, normal nerve transmission from motor nerves to striated muscle is interrupted. This disease primarily affects the muscles of the eyes, esophagus, and respiratory muscles, as well as the extremities [1]. The total prevalence of MG is 15 – 20 per 100.000 persons and an estimated 15 – 20% of all MG develop a myasthenic crisis in their course of disease [34].

Conservative therapies are thymectomy and administration of cholinesterase-blocking substances [35]. In cases with severe progression, immunosuppressives are also given to suppress autoantibody synthesis. TPE has implemented with good results, especially in the case of severe, previously therapy-resistant progression. The rapid elimination of autoantibodies achieved with TPE results in an improvement in clinical symptoms within hours to days (36). With the rapid improvement in the symptoms of their patients through TPE, Johnson et al. observed no increased tendency towards infection as a result of immunoglobulin elimination [37].

The rationale for TA is to remove circulating autoantibodies. In acute attacks, TA is the first-line therapy (Table 1). The seropositve and seronegative patients respond to TPE. TPE most uses in myasthenic crisis and perioperatively for thymectomy, or as an adjunct to other therapies to maintain optimal clinical status [10]. TPE works rapidly, the clinical effect can be seen within 24 hours or longer. The benefits will likely subside in 2 – 4 weeks, if immunosuppressive therapies are not initiated to keep antibody levels from reforming [10]. TPE and IA are the first-line methods for treating a MG crisis [36]. There are some retrospective and comparative studies of both of these approaches [34, 38 - 40]. A combination of TA and immunosuppressives seems to be successful but randomized trials are necessary.

Multiple Sclerosis (MS)

MS is a replasing, remitting chronic demyelinating disease of the CNS and is the most common cause of neurologic disability in young adults [41]. It has estimated that some 120,000 to 140,000 patients are affected by MS alone in Germany. Worldwide, there are more than one million afflicted with the disease, and in the United States alone, there are more than 300,000 patients. MS is also diagnosed in children and adolescents. Estimates suggest that 8,000-10,000 children (up to 18 years old) in the United States have MS, and another 10,000-15,000 have experienced at least one symptom suggestive of MS.

The definition of MS as an autoimmune disease is based on the following characteristics [23]:

- HLA association and genetic predisposition: T cell subset and cytokine correlation with disease activity,
- clinical responses to immunosuppression and immune activators,
- analogies with experimental autoimmune encephalomyelitis,
- cero spinal fluid oligoclonal IgG bands,
- CNS pathology using immunocytochemistry techniques,
- evidence of intrathecal synthesis of tumor necrosis factor beta in MS, and the level of TNF alpha in cerebro-spinal fluid may correlate with the severity and progression of disease and reflect histologic disease activity in MS,
- increased levels of gamma interferon correlate with the disease worsening [23]

The rationale for treating MS patients with TA derives from the presence of these circulating antimyelin antibodies, non-antibody demyelinating factors, aquaporin-4-specific serum autoantibodies, and neuroelectric blocking factors (Table 1) [42, 43]. TPE removes antibodies and other humoral factors from the circulation safely and effectively. TPE has also been shown to increase the number and percentage of suppressor T cells and decrease the helper T cells in MS patients, thus effectively decreasing the ratio of elevated helper/inducer to suppressor/cytotoxic cell. This point is important, because T cells play a pivotal role in the pathogenesis of MS [1]. Children should treated with corticosteroids. If corticosteroids alone do not bring enough improvement, other treatments, including IVIG, Interferon ß 1a, rituximab, and TPE and IA are available to treat-to-treat MS attacks. Especially in steroid refractory MS relapse immunoadsorption was found by Schimrigk et al. and Lipphardt to be effective and well tolerated [44, 45]. In 147 patients Schimrigk et al. found in 74,4% an improved functionally after a mean of 5.4 IA treatments within 7 – 10 days.

In the guidelines of the AAC of the ASFA the acute MS has the category II and The RG 1B and the chronic MS the category III with the RG 2B [9, 10]. But the physicians should make individual decisions on the suitable of TA as the treatment for their patients with MS [46].

Pediatric Autoimmune Neuropsychiatric Disorders Associated with Streptococcal Infections (PANDAS); Sydenham's Chorea (SC)

PANDAS and Sydenham's chorea are postinfectious neuropsychiatric disorders. Both of neuropsychiatric symptoms, which typically follow Group-A beta-hemolytic streptococcus (GABHS) infection, and may have shared etiopathogenesis. Postulated pathogenesis suggests that streptococcal antigens induce antineural antibodies by an abnormal immune response [10, 47]. GABHS infection has associated with childhood-onset neuropsychiatric disorders, such as, obsessive-compulsive disorder and tic disorders. The onset of PANDAS is acute and dramatic, presenting with emotional/mood lability, attention deficit, deterioration of handwriting, separation anxiety, tactile/sensory defensiveness, enuresis, cognitive deficits, and motor hyperactivity [10].

Sydenham's chorea is the main common acquired chorea of childhood. The major clinical manifestations are chorea, hypotonia, and emotional lability. The duration of SC is several months with a recurrence rate of about 20 percent [10]. Choreatic movements are rapid, jerky, and involuntary and affect the face, trunk, and extremitites. The mean ages of onset for PANDAS and SC are 6.8 years and 8.4 years old, respectively. SC is diagnosed exclusively by clinical presentations and a history of rheumatic fever. Although PANDAS is temporally associated with GABHS, it is not associated with rheumatic fever. Laboratory tests show elevated or increasing streptococcal antibody titers, but an elevated titer does not necessarily indicate a recent streptococal infection. In PANDAS, the presence of streptococcal infection is associated with at least two episodes of neuropsychiatric symptoms as well as negative throat culture or stable titers during times of remission [10].

The treatments for PANDAS include antibotics and cognitive behavioral therapy. Severe form of SC is treated with diazepam, valproic acid, carbamazepine, or haloperidol [9]. If these fail, corticosteroids may be tried. While children with SC require long-term penicillin prophylaxis to reduce the risk of rheumatic carditis, the efficacy of penicillin prohylaxis in preventing symptom exacerbations in children with PANDAS remains doubtful. In symptomatic or refractory patients with PANDAS or SC, IVIG (1 g/kg/day for 2 days) or TPE has shown to reduce symptom severity or shorten the course. In the guidelines on the use of TA from the AAC of the ASFA PANDAS or SC have the category I with RG 1B (Table 1) [10]. The first-line treatments include corticosteroids, IVIG, and therapeutic apheresis for severe diseases agents such as rituximab or cyclophosphamide are used [48]:

Chronic Focal Encephalitis (CFE) (Rasmussen Encephalitis, RE)

The CFE is a chronic encephalitis characterized by intractable focal seizures and slowly progressive neurological deterioration was originally described in 3 patients by Rasmussen in 1958 [9]. Onset is typically in childhood with a mean age 6.8 ± 5.1 years but a similar syndrome has described in adults, too. The etiology is unknown. Antecedent infection with Epstein-Barr virus, herpes simplex, enterovirus, or cytomegalovirus has implicated. In three adult patients with RE, Cytomegalo-virus genome has been found in resected cortical tissue. Other investigations such as cerebrospinal fluid analysis are typically normal, only mild lymphocytic pleocytosis and elevated protein may found. The hallmark of RE is epilepsy uncontrollable with anticonvulsant drugs, progressive hemiparesis, and progressive unilateral cerebral atrophy. There is progressive loss of function in the affected cerebral hemisphere and cognitive decline [10]. Anticonvulsants are necessary but are not always effective in controlling the disease nor do they stop its progression. Subtotal, functional complete hemispherectomy can markedly reduce seizure activity in a majority of patients but results in permanent contralateral hemiplegia corticosteroids and IVIG given for up to two years in a tapering schedule to diminish epilepsy and other symptoms. Patients with RE and antibodies against neural molecules, and auto-antibodies can be produced in the CNS after cytotoxic T cell-mediated neuronal damage [10]. The CFE has the category III and RG 2 C for TPE and IA in the AAC of the ASFA (Table 1) [10]:

Neuropsychological assessment may be helpful in evaluating patients with slowly progressive disease to determine whether TPE is effective in postponing surgical therapy. An initial course of TPE may followed by 2 days of IVIG 1 g/kg/day. Monthly IA of 1.5 – 2 TPV per treatment has been reported effective in one patient [10]. Confirmation of anti-GluR3 antibodies may support the use of TA in patients with Rasmussen´s encephalitis.

Other Neurological Diseases

Other neurological diseases have also been treated with TA. *Acute disseminated encephalomyopathy (ADEM)* is an acute inflammatory monophasic demyelinating disease that affects the brain and spinal cord, which typically occurs after a febrile, viral prodrome or vaccination [9, 49]. The pathogenesis is perhaps a disseminated multifocal inflammation and patchy demyelination associated with a transient autoimmune response against myelin or other autoantigenes. The typical symptom is that of multifocal neurological deficits such as ataxia, weakness, dysarthria, and dysphagia accompanied by change in mental status. Most commonly, it is a monophasic illness that lasts from 2 to 4 weeks. Predominantly children and young adults are affected. The differentiation of ADEM from the first attack of multiple sclerosis has prognostic and therapeutic implications. ADEM has these features which help to distinguish it from MS: florid polysymptomatic presentation, lack of oligoclonal band in CSF, predominance of MRI lesions in the subcortical region with relative sparing of the periventricular area, and complete or partial resolution of MRI lesions during convalescence [10].

Corticosteroids are the first-line therapy, which hasten recovery and result in clinical improvement in up to 60 percent of patients. IVIG is for patients who do not respond to corticosteroids [10]. TPE is used and has a clearly defined role in other neurological conditions that are presumed to be immunologically mediated. TPE removes presumed offending antibodies as well as through immunomodulation. The category II for TPE with the RG 2C after the AAC of the ASFA is assigned on paucity of data [9, 10] (Table 1).

Lambert-Eaton myasthenic syndrome is a rare, but reasonably well-understood, antibody-mediated autoimmune disease that is caused by serum auto-antibodies and results in muscle weakness and autonomic dysfunction [50]. Like MG, Lambert-Eaton syndrome is based on a disorder of the transmission of neuromuscular excitation. In this case no acetylcholine is released.

Miller-Fisher syndrome (MFS) is characterized by the acute onset of ophthalmoplegia, ataxia, and areflexia. It is considered to be a variant form of Guillain-Barré syndrome. Because MFS is classified as a variant form of GBS and has a close association with the presence of the anti-GQ1b antibody, one would expect the efficacy of treatment with TPE or IVIG to have been proved [1].

Stiff-Man syndrome (SMS) is a rare neurological disease caused by autoantibodies to GABAergic neurons [1, 51]. Various authors reported that TPE might be beneficial for the management of patients with SMS for acute exacerbations or long-term maintenance [51 - 53]. TPE is well tolerated with low adverse events.

Other neurological diseases, such as cryoglobulinemic polyneuropathy, central nervous system systemic lupus, acquired neuromyotonia, polymyositis/dermatomyositis, polyneuropathy in paraproteinemia, neuropathy by hyperlipidemia, and encephalopathy in metabolic/hematologic diseases such as thyrotoxicosis, hepatic coma, and M. Moschcowitz are diseases that involve more organ systems and are mentioned elsewhere. Extensive blood and plasma exchange for the treatment of the coagulopathy have been successfully implemented in children with meningococcemia [54]. In the neurological diseases mentioned above, TA can be regarded as a support therapy to the current treatment strategies.

CONCLUSION

All mentioned TA methods are still technically complicated and very expensive. The costs of the mentioned TA methods varied widely for example in Germany, the costs are for TPE between 830 and 1,620 €, and for IA between 2,040 and 2,240 € per treatment [55]. It is the task of the manufactures to develop simpler and less costly techniques.

Physicians are committed for helping all patients entrusted to them to the best of their knowledge and this means that medical treatment- and particularly the apheresis processes must become affordable. This demand represents a great challenge to physicians, politicians, health organisations and, above all, to the manufacturers. Industry constantly justifies the high costs with the extensive research and development required. All those involved in the healthcare system must intensify their cooperation in this respect.

The prognosis of immunological diseases such as Goodpasture syndrome or myasthenia gravis with their varying organ manifestations has improved considerably in recent years due to very aggressive therapy schemes. These include therapeutic apheresis in combination with immunosuppressive therapies and/or biologic agents. In mild form of autoimmune disease, immunosuppressive therapies and/or biologic agents seem to be sufficient. In these cases, therapeutic apheresis must combined with an immunosuppressive therapy and/or biologic agent. Use of newer technologies, such as immunoadsorption, possible in combination with recent biologics, might offer some new perspectives for extracorporeal treatment of immunological diseases.

But for all mentioned diseases the quotient relevant for cost – effectivity assessment (cost of treatment – cost saved): (improvement in life quality) must be discussed and calculated exactly by all involvement persons. After Malchesky every effort should be made to delay the progression of chronic diseases. TA is clearly an important tool in treatment of many complex conditions now and in the future [56].

REFERENCES

[1] Bambauer R, Latza R, Schiel R. *Therapeutic Plasma Exchange and Selective Plasma Separation Method.* Fundamental Technologies,

Pathology and Clinical Results. Pabst Science Publishers, Lengerich, Germany, 2013.

[2] Hafer C, Golla P, Gericke M et al. Membrane versus centrifuge-based therapeutic plasma exchange: a randomized prospective crossover study. *Int Urol Nephrol.* 2015, Doi.1007/s11255-015-1137-3.

[3] Klein J, Horejsi V (eds.) Immunology. *Thieme Verlag,* Stuttgart, New York, 1997.

[4] Dunkley M, Pabst R, Crips A. An important role for intestinally derived T cells in respiratory defence. *Immunol Today.* 1997;16:231-8.

[5] Lang B, Newsom-Davis J, Wray D et al. Autoimmune aetiology for myasthenic (Eaton-Lambert) syndrome. *Lancet* 1981;II:224-6.

[6] Snyder HW, Balint JP, Jones FR. Modulation of immunity in patients with autoimmune disease and cancer treated by extracorporeal immunoadsorption with Prosorba® columns. *Sem Hematol* 1989;26:31-41.

[7] Bambauer R, R Schiel, B Lehmann, C Bambauer. Therapeutic apheresis, technical overview. *ARPN J Sci Technol.* 2012;2:399-421. Available from: http://www.ejournalofscience.org/archive/vol2no5/vol2no5_1. pdf. Accessed July 22, 2013.

[8] Bambauer R, C Bambauer, R Latza, R. Schiel. Therapeutic apheresis in nephrology. *Clin Nephrol Urol Sci.* 2014; http://www.hoajonline.com/journals/pdf/2054-7161-1-2.pdf. doi: 10.7243/2054-7161-1-2.

[9] Schwartz J, Winters J, Padmanabhan L et al. Guidelines on the Use of Therapeutic Apheresis in Clinical Practice-Evidence-Based Approach from the Writing Committee of the American Society for Apheresis: The Sixth Special Issue. *J Clin Apher.* 2013;28:145-284.

[10] Schwartz J, Padmanabhan, Aqui N et al. Guidelines on the Use of Therapeutic Apheresis in Clinical Practice – Evidence-Based Approach from the Writing Committee of the American Society for Apheresis: The Seventh Special Issue. *J Clin Apher.* 2016;31:149-338.

[11] Agishi T, Kaneko J, Hasuo Y et al. Double filtration plasmapheresis with no or minimal amount of blood derivate for substitution. In:

Plasma Exchange, H. G. Sieberth (Ed.), *Schattauer, Stuttgart,* Germany, 1980; p. 53-57.

[12] Yamamoto A, Kawaguchi A, Harada-Shiba M et al. Apheresis technology for prevention and regression of atherosclerosis: an overview. *Ther Apher.* 1997;1(3):233–241.

[13] Klingel R, Mausfeld P, Fassbender C et al. Lipidfiltration—safe and effective methodology to perform lipid-apheresis. *Transfus Apher Sci.* 2004; 30(3):245–254.

[14] Stoffel W, Borberg H, Greve V. Application of specific extracorporeal removal of low density lipoprotein in familial hypercholesterolemia. *Lancet* II:1981:1005-1007.

[15] Shelat SG. Practical considerations for planning a therapeutic apheresis procedure. *Am J Med* 2010;123:777-84.

[16] Ariga T, Yu RK. Antiglycolipid antibodies in Guillain-Barré syndrome and related diseases. Review of clinical features and antibody specifities. *J Neurosci Res* 2005;80:1-17.

[17] Meneses de Oliveira FT, De Luca NC, Tilbery CP. Plasmapheresis therapy for immune-mediated diseases in neurology: literature review. *Glon Vac Immunol.* 2016;1(2):29-32.

[18] Miller AC, Rashid RM, Sinert RH. Guillain-Barré Syndrome. EMedicine specialities >Emergency Medicine> *Neurology update* Apr 23. 2010). 792008-overview.

[19] Weinstein R. Is there a scientific rationale for therapeutic plasma exchange or intravenous immune globulins in the treatment of acute Guillain-Barré syndrome? *J Clin Apher* 1995;10:150-7.

[20] Weinstein R. Therapeutic apheresis in neurological disorders: a survey of the evidence in support of current category I and II indications for therapeutic plasma exchange. *J Clin Apher. 2008;*23: 196-201.

[21] Korintenberg R, Schessl J, Kirchner J et al. Intravenous administered immunoglobulin in the treatment of childhood Guillain-Barré-syndrome: A randomized trial. *Pediatrics* 2005;116:8-16.

[22] Kleymann I, Branagan TH. Treatment of chronic Inflammatory Demyelinating Polyneuropathy. *Nerve Muscle.* 2015;15:47-55.

[23] Khatri BO. Therapeutic apheresis in neurologic disorders. *Ther Apher.* 1999;3:161-71.
[24] Dada MA, Kaplan AA. Plasmapheresis treatment in Guillain-Barré-syndrome. Potential benefit over IVIG in patients with axonal involvement. *Ther Apher Dial.* 2004;8:409-12.
[25] Haupt WF, Birkmann C, van der Ven G. Apheresis and selective adsorption plus immunoglobulin treatment in Guillain-Barré syndrome. *Ther Apher.* 2000;4:198-200.
[26] Lin JH, Tu KH, Chang CH et al. Prognostic factors and complication rates for double-filtration plasmapheresis in patients with Guillain-Barré syndrome. *Transf Apher Sci.* 2015;52(1):78-83.
[27] Mühlhausen J, Kitze B, Huppke P et al. Apheresis treatment of acute inflammatory demyelinating disorders. *Atheroscler Suppl.* 2015;18:251-256.
[28] Prajapati P, Dighe M, Kothari F. Role of therapeutic plasma exchange in neuro-immunological Disorder. *Int J Res Med.* 2018;7(2):15-18.
[29] Ryan M, Ryan SJ. Chronic inflammatory demyelinating polyneuropathy: Considerations for diagnosis, management, and population health. *Am J Managed Care.* 2018;24(17):S371-S378.
[30] Allen D, Giannopoulos K, Gray I et al. Antibodies to peripheral nerve myelin proteins in chronic inflammatory demyelinating polyradiculoneuropathy. *J Peripher Berv Syst.* 2005;10:174-80.
[31] Hughes RAC, Bouche P, Cornblatt DR et al. European Federation of Neurological Societies/Peripheral Nerve Society guideline on management of chronic inflammatory demyelinating polyradiculoneuropathy: report of a joint task force of the European of Neurological Societies and the Peripheral nerve Society. *Europ J Neurol.* 2006;13:326-34.
[32] Beydoun SR, Brannagan TH, Donofrino P et al. Chronic inflammatory demyelinating polyradiculoneuropathy 101-pitfalls and perls of diagnosis and treatment. *US Neurology* 2017;13(1):18-25.
[33] Tselmin S, Julius U, Bornstein SR, Hohenstein B. Low rate infectious complications following immunoadsorption therapy without regular

substitution of intravenous immunoglobulins. *Atheroscleros Suppl.* 2017;30:278-282.

[34] Schroeter M, Thayssen G, Kaiser J. Myasthenia Gravis – exacerbation and crisis. *Neurol Int Open.* 2018;2(1):E10-E15.

[35] Bachmann K, Burkhardt D, Schreitert J et al. Thymectomy is more effective than conservative treatment for myasthenia gravis regarding outcome and clinical improvement. *Surgery* 2009;145:392-8.

[36] Ebadi H, Barth D, Bril V: Safety of plasma exchange therapy in patients with myasthenia gravis. *Muscle Nerve* 2013;47:510-4. doi: 10.1002/mus.23626.

[37] Johnson RB, Muder RR, Spyros SD et al. Staphylococcal carriage and infection in myasthenia gravis patients receiving therapeutic apheresis. *J Clin Apher.* 1988;4:155-7.

[38] Alemam AI, Abdlulrahmean AI. Seropositivity in Myasthenia gravis as a predictor of response to therapeutic plasma exchange. *J Neurol Res.* 2019;9(1-2):8-13.

[39] Negi G, Ahuja R, Gupta V. Et al. Therapeutic plasma exchange: A study of indications and efficacy. *Glob J Transfus Med.* 2018;8(2):136-139.

[40] Usmani A, Kwan L, Wahib-Khalil D, et al. Excellent response to therapeutic plasma exchange in myasthenia gravis patients irrespective of antibody status. *J Clin Apher.* 2019, https://doi.org/10.1002/jca.21694.

[41] Flachenecker P, Zettl UK. Epidemiologie. In: Schmidt RM, Hoffmann F (eds.). Multiple Sklerose. *Urban + Fischer*, München, 2006, p 11-7.

[42] Khatri BO. Therapeutic apheresis in multiple sclerosis and other central nervous system disorders. *Ther Apher.* 2000;4:263-70.

[43] Magana SM, Pittcock SJ, Lennon VA et al. NMO-IgG status in fulminant inflammatory CNS demyelinating disorders. *Arch Neurol.* 2009;66:964-6.

[44] Schimrigk S, Faiss J, Köhler W. Escalation therapy of steroid refractory multiple sclerosis relapse with Tryptophan Immunoadsorption – Observational multicenter study with 147 patients. *Eur Neurol.* 2016;75:300-306.

[45] Lipphardt M, Mühlhausen J, Kitze B et al. Immunoadsorption or plasma exchange in steroid-refractory multiple sclerosis and neuromyelitis optica. *J Clin Apher.* 2019. https://doi.org/10.1002/jca.21686.

[46] Haaris ES, Meiselman HJ, Moriarty PM. Therapeutic plasma exchange for the treatment of systemic sclerosis: A comprehensive review and analysis. *J Sagepub Com.* 2018, https://doi.org/10.1177/2397198318758606.

[47] Calaprice D, Tona J, Parker-Hill EC et al. A survey of pediatric acute onset neuropsychiatric syndrome characteristics and course. *J Child Adolesc Psychopharmacology.* 2017;(27(7):607-618.

[48] Nosadini M, Sarori S, Sharma S et al. Immunotherapeutics in pediatric autoimmune central nervous system disease: Agents and Mechanisms. *Sem Pediat Neurol.* 2017;24(3):214-228.

[49] Longoni G, Levy DM, Yeh EA. The changing landscape of childhood inflammatory central nervous system disorders. *J Pediatrics.* 2016;(179):24-32e2.

[50] Vershuuren JGM, Wirtz PW, Titulaer MJ et al. Available treatment options for the management of Lambert-Eaton myasthenic syndrome. *Exp Opin Pharmacothera.* 2006;7:1323-36.

[51] Shariatmadar S, Noto TA. Plasma exchange in Stiff-Man syndrome, *Ther Apher.* 2001;5(1): https://doi.org/10.1046/j.1526-0968.2001.005001064.x

[52] Pagano MB, Murinson BB, Tobian AAR, King KE. Efficacy of therapeutic plasma exchange for treatment of stiff-person syndrome. *Transfusion.* 2014;54(1): https://doi.org/10.1111/trf.12573.

[53] Albahra S, Yates SG, Joseph D et al. Role of plasma exchange in stiff person syndrome. *Transf Apher Sci.* 2019. hhtps://doi.org/10.1016/j.transci.2019.03.015.

[54] Churchwell KB, Mc Manus ML, Kent P et al. Intensive blood and plasma exchange for treatment of coagulopathy in meningococcemia. *J Clin Apher* 1995;10:171-7.

[55] Kribben A, Lütkes P, Müller H. Costs calculation for dialysis and other therapy methods in nephrology. *Das Krankenhaus* 2004;5:356-63.
[56] Malchesky PS. Therapeutic Apheresis: Why? *Ther Apher Dial.* 2015;19(5):417-26. doi: 10.111/1744-9987:12353.

In: Neurological Diseases
Editor: Philip L. Thygesen

ISBN: 978-1-53616-205-9
© 2019 Nova Science Publishers, Inc.

Chapter 2

POSSIBLE THERAPEUTIC EFFECTS OF CEFTRIAXONE IN ALUMINUM NEUROTOXICITY WHEN APPLIED BEFORE AND AFTER ALUMINUM

Ankica Jelenković[1,*]*, Marina D. Jovanović*[2]*,*
Ivana Stevanović[2] *and Vera Prokić*[2]

[1]University of Belgrade, Institute for Biological Research
"Siniša Stanković", Belgrade, Republic of Serbia
[2]Military Medical Academy, University of Defense,
Institute for Medical Research, Belgrade, Republic of Serbia

ABSTRACT

Ceftriaxone, a β-lactam antibiotic primarily applied for its antimicrobial effects, in the last decade was suggested to be neuroprotective as well due to its abilities to increase the expression of membrane-bound glutamate transporter EAAT2/GLT-1 and counteract

---

[*] Corresponding Author's E-mail: jelaka@yahoo.com.

glutamate-mediated neurotoxicity. The dysfunction of GLT-1 transporter and the consequent accumulation of excessive extracellular glutamate is correlated with multiple neurodegenerative pathologies. Oxidative stress, one of the multifold and complex variables responsible for the development of these diseases, is also recognized in aluminum neurotoxicity. Furthermore, aluminum has almost unambiguously been shown to take part in the etiopathogenetic processes of Alzheimer's and other neurodegenerative diseases. Due to all the previously mentioned facts, it was of interest to examine whether ceftriaxone could influence the aluminum brain neurotoxic effects. To do so, we subjected four groups of adult male Wistar rats to four different treatments *via* stereotaxic brain surgery. Saline and aluminum chloride (3.7×10^{-4} g/kg) were applied intrahippocampally. Aluminium was given prior to, as well as after five consecutive days of ceftriaxone treatment (200mg/kg body weight, applied intraperitoneally). Rats were decapitated on the 13th day of recovery after surgery. In the four brain regions (forebrain cortex, striatum, basal forebrain and hippocampus) the activity of cytochrome c oxidase and glucose-6-phosphate dehydrogenase were determined, as well as the level of reduced glutathione. Based on the obtained results, it was evident that ceftriaxone significantly attenuated the detrimental effects of aluminum on all of the analyzed brain parameters, but also it restored them entirely. Besides, ceftriaxone pre-treatment displayed stronger effects than the after-treatment. Accordingly, the ability of ceftriaxone to alleviate the harmful protoxidative effects of aluminum in the brain can be a new approach to combating oxidative stress that is involved in the pathogenesis of various brain disorders.

Keywords: ceftriaxone, aluminum, neurotoxicity, oxidative stress, neurodegenerative diseases

ABBREVIATIONS

AMPA	alfa-amino-3-hydroxy-5-methyl-4-isoxazoleproprionic acid
ATP	adenosine triphosphate
Aβ	amyloid β
BFb	basal forebrain
DNA	deoxyribonucleic acid
EAAC	excitatory amino acid carrier

EAAT	excitatory amino acid transporter
FbC	forebrain cortex
GABA	γ-aminobutyric acid
GFAP	glial fibrillary acidic protein
GLAST	glutamate-aspartate transporter
GLT-1	glutamate transporter 1
H	hippocampus
ip	intraperitoneally
NMDA	N-methyl-D-aspartate
S	striatum
SOD	superoxide dismutase

INTRODUCTION

Beta-lactams, a class of broad-spectrum antimicrobials, still now remains one of the most important groups of antibiotics. They are currently clinically used very much, most widely of all antimicrobial classes of drugs. They are widely prescribed for the prevention and treatment of bacterial infections.

Although the pharmacological properties among these agents vary, they are well distributed throughout the body with a sufficiently high concentration for therapeutic purposes. In the last couple of decades it has become obvious that beta-lactam antibiotics could reach the brain after penetrating the blood–brain barrier. Furthermore, they exhibit certain therapeutic effects in neurodegenerative disorders, at least under experimental conditions. This is the result of a great spectrum of research conducted by Rothstein et al. [1]. Due to their almost revolutionary discovery, it has become quite clear that these drugs, besides their accepted antibacterial properties, also have a completely different mechanism of action. Indeed, their ability to reduce the concentration of glutamate in the synaptic cleft and generally extracellularly, which consequently reduces the probability of glutamate excitotoxicity, was observed. Based on this mechanism of action, it was assumed that beta-lactam antibiotics, including ceftriaxone, may act against the diseases of the central nervous system known as neurodegenerative diseases where, at least in part, glutamate toxicity has been proven: "The chronic inhibition of glutamate uptake produces a model of slow neurotoxicity" [2].

Despite the increased prevalence of patients suffering from neurodegenerative and mental diseases, pharmacological agents currently available for the curative or disease-modifying actions are extremely modest. Their treatment is directed only to symptomatic and supportive care. Thus, the current information concerning the effects of beta lactams is very attractive for a wide range pathophysiological modulation of these diseases. The discovery of Rothstein et al. resulted in a number of research studies focused on the effects of beta-lactam antibiotics in different cell lines and animal models of neurodegenerative diseases, as well as in people suffering from some of these diseases.

A substantial amount of evidence pointed out the neurotoxicological potential of aluminum, both in animals and in humans as well. A great number of studies strongly proposed association between aluminum and brain aging and its participation in the etiopathogenesis of neurodegenerative diseases, such as Alzheimer's, Parkinson's and Huntington's disease and multiple sclerosis, all of which are very complex, and genetically, environmentally, and lifestyle determined [3]. The exact molecular mechanism underlying the aluminum toxicity remains unclear, which is quite expected when it is known that aluminum "influences more than 200 biologically important reactions" [4]. Due to its multifaceted targets and readiness for binding to different biological molecules, the neurotoxicity of aluminum could lead to an extraordinarily large number of brain biochemical and structural changes, and also to neurobehavioral disturbances as well. Among other disturbances, the disruption of essential metal homeostasis, oxidative stress and oxidative protein modification are documented in neurological disorders associated with aluminum overload. Furthermore, it was already postulated that neurotoxic effects of aluminum could be mediated, among other mechanisms, by the elevation of excitatory amino acid glutamate in the brain [5].

Aluminum accounts for 8.6% of the earth crust. In the developing countries it has been widely used as a purifying agent, for tableware, food packaging, in food products, even in the off-the-shelf infant formulas, in adjuvants and medicines, such as antacids, phosphate binders, buffered aspirins, vaccines, as well as in the cosmetic industry [6]. Workers in aluminum production and aluminum user industries, as well as aluminum welders, are widely exposed to aluminum and its compounds. The exposure to aluminum occurs through air, food and water, including inhalation, ingestion, and dermal contact, which could, in the long run, accumulate in biological systems. All the aforementioned uses of aluminum lead to an easy and extensive exposure of humans to aluminum in their daily life. Altered renal function leads to a more pronounced susceptibility to aluminum toxicity due to its insufficient elimination and consequent accumulation in different organs including the brain, thus leading to their dysfunction. Therefore, in terms of human health risk, aluminum displays a general public health hazard [7].

The accumulation of excess extracellular glutamate and subsequent overstimulation of glutamatergic receptors, the prominent mechanism of aluminum activity, requires suppression in order to prevent its harmful effects. Based on the first findings of Rothstein et al., concerning the ceftriaxone effects on glutamate transporters and the consequential reduction of glutamate extracellular concentration and neuroprotection [1], the focus of this chapter will be the current study undertaken to determine the efficacy of ceftriaxone in aluminum toxicity, expressed biochemically in certain brain structures of rats which were intrahippocampally treated with aluminum chloride.

GLUTAMATE HOMEOSTASIS IN THE BRAIN

Glutamate is the principal excitatory amino acid neurotransmitter in the mammalian central nervous system, since nearly all excitatory neurons are glutamatergic and more than 40% of all brain synapses are estimated to be glutamatergic. In cases of excessive extracellular amounts or longer periods of action, glutamate can also be a potential neurotoxin. Together with GABA, the most abundant inhibitory neurotransmitter, it is essential in regulating many aspects of brain functions that are based on quite complex signaling. As the result of an action potential, glutamatergic neurons release glutamate into extracellular space (glutamatergic synapse) *via* exocytosis that participates in the signaling process through the stimulation of two different types of glutamatergic postsynaptic receptors - metabotropic and ionotropic receptors (NMDA and AMPA), which modulate the synaptic activity and plasticity. The ionotropic group of receptors is considered to be mainly responsible for excitotoxicity.

The action of glutamate being released into the synaptic cleft must be terminated and the excess glutamate must be rapidly removed from the synaptic cleft in order to avoid its high concentrations in synapses, the overstimulation of glutamate receptors and consequent toxic effects, due to the fact that extracellular glutamate should be low in physiological conditions.

The termination of glutamate neurotransmission is achieved by its uptake into neurons and surrounding glial cells *via* specific transporters in high-affinity sodium-dependent and energy (ATP) consumption reactions. In short, neurotransmission involves biosynthesis, storage, release, interaction with receptor(s) and inactivation of the neurotransmitter. The role of transporters is to rapidly remove glutamate from synaptic cleft and to maintain its stimulatory, but not toxic levels within synapses. They are expressed (in some cells in high densities) in neuronal and glial cell membrane (astrocytes, microglia, and oligodendrocytes). The clearance of the extracellular glutamate can be achieved in three different ways, wherein the glutamate is distributed into three compartments:

- the uptake into the postsynaptic neurons,
- the re-uptake into the presynaptic neurons, and
- the uptake into a nonneuronal, glial compartment.

Postsynaptic neurons remove only a little glutamate. The active re-uptake into the presynaptic neurons could be significant in some circumstances. The first two mechanisms of glutamate uptake appear to be less important than astrocytic transport and they are not sufficient to replenish the neuronal glutamate that was released.

The glutamate transport function of astrocytes is one of the most important ones in glutamate homeostasis, i.e., the balance between glutamate release and elimination. The astrocytes are distributed throughout the grey and the white matter of the brain and the spinal cord. In addition to being glutamate transporters, astrocytes possess a wide variety of other transporters, receptors and signaling molecules, all of which are a part of fundamental processes responsible for regulating the equilibrium in the central nervous system. Astrocytes are as well as an essential component of the blood–brain barrier.

The failure of proper removal of glutamate from the synaptic cleft inevitably leads to sustained elevation and excessive accumulation of extracellular glutamate levels with an over-stimulation of glutamatergic receptors. This has a profound impact on brain functions and can result in a number of pathological conditions. The glutamate (mediated) excitotoxicity is a result of the cascade of calcium-dependent enzymatic pathway activation with a consequent dysfunction of calcium homeostasis, mitochondrial action and failure of energy production, an increased production of reactive oxygen/nitrogen species (free radicals) and the development of oxidative and nitrosative stress. These disorders are all implicated in the pathogenesis of neurodegeneration, which is the terminal effect of the cumulative loss in structure or function of neurons. So far, glutamate-mediated toxicity has been targeted at least in two ways, by NMDAR antagonists and by compounds that target calcium influx. However, the protective effects obtained under experimental conditions are far from the desired clinical usage.

Glutamate Transporters and Termination of Glutamate Neurotransmitter Activity

Glutamate homeostasis is tightly regulated by the interplay between the glutamate release and glutamate clearance. The essential place in these processes belongs to glutamate transporters. They mediate the cellular uptake (transport) of L-glutamate, L-aspartate and D-aspartate into the cytosol of different cells.

The crucial role of glutamate transporters is in terminating glutamatergic transmission and in maintaining its optimal extracellular concentration that is essential for the preservation of neuronal physiological functions and their survival. On the other hand, the recycled glutamate is the source of its regeneration, a primary precondition for its repeated release. Thus, glutamate transporters are the key players in both health and disease.

Glutamate transporters are proteins expressed in the plasma membrane of different cells and in synaptic vesicles in glutamatergic neurons [8]. Mitochondrial glutamate transmembrane carriers have also recently been discovered. The localization of transporters in the brain is complex and varies widely in their expression pattern in individual cells (cell-specific expression), as well as in brain regions [9]. Predominantly, the expression in some cells means that they also exist at the same time on the membrane of other cell types, but only to a lesser extent.

So far, several families that transport glutamate have been identified:

- the plasma membrane excitatory amino acid transporters (EAATs)
- the glutamate-cysteine antiporter (exchanger), and
- the vesicular glutamate transporters (VGLUTs).

The family of EAATs (glutamate transporters) belongs to the SLC1 family. The glutamate/amino acid solute carrier (SLC) transporters are a group of more than 400 membrane-bound proteins organized into 65 families. They are localized on the plasma membrane, as well as on the membranes of various subcellular organelles of different cells. These proteins facilitate the transport of diverse substrates across biological membranes, such as the inorganic ions, amino acids, lipids, neurotransmitters, drugs, etc.

The excitatory amino acid transporters provide the only known endogenous mechanism for the clearance of extracellular glutamate in mammals. They consist of five structurally different human and rat subtypes that have already been cloned (EAAT1-5) [10]. Three of them were identified in the rat brain, which also have human homologues (rat/human homolog): GLAST corresponds to human EAAT1, GLT-1 to EAAT2 and EAAC1 to EAAT3. The two other human and rodent brain subtypes of transporters, EAAT4 and EAAT5, share common nomenclature.

The predominant and the most abundant glutamate transporter subtype in the adult brain is GLT-1/EAAT2, also known as solute carrier family 1 member 2 (SLC1A2). This protein is encoded by the *SLC1A2* gene in humans. GLT-1/EAAT2 is primarily, but not exclusively, expressed at high densities on astroglial cells throughout the brain and spinal cord (not in neurons). They play a central role in the maintenance of the extracellular glutamate homeostasis, accounting for more than 90% of glutamate transporter activity in the brain [11, 12]. Together with GLAST/EAAT1, they represent the primary transport carriers for glutamate uptake into astrocytes. The surface of the astrocyte processes is predominantly the GLAST/EAAT1 expression site, known as the solute carrier family 1 member 3 (SLC1A3). Such localization of transporters physically brings them closer to the synaptic cleft from which they uptake the released glutamate.

EAAT1, as well as EAAT3 (SLC1A1) are expressed in the neuronal cell bodies and dendrites. EAAT4 (SLC1A6) is expressed almost exclusively in cerebellar Purkinje cells, while EAAT5 (SLC1A7) is expressed predominantly in the retina where it suppresses the transmitter release from the presynaptic terminal [13]. EAAT3 and EAAT4 are expressed in the postsynaptic neurons (often GABAergic). EAAT4 and EAAT5 are expressed in the vestibular hair cells.

The effects of plasma membrane glutamate transporters are regulated at multiple levels:

- the expression of transporter proteins,
- the activities (biochemical and functional) of the expressed transporters,
- the membrane localization of transporters, which affects their activation/inhibition.

Among the other glutamate transporter proteins, there are also those specialized for transporting the amino acids across the plasma membranes. They are located in the cell membrane, predominantly in astrocytes, but also in neurons, oligodendrocytes and microglia [14]. One of them is the system x_c^-, an antiporter of cystine and glutamate that works as a glutamate-cystine exchanger. The glutamate-cystine antiporter belongs to the solute carrier family and SLC7 is the family of amino acid transporters. This antiporter contains the subunits of xCT (also known as solute carrier family 7 member 11, SLC7A11) and SLC3A2. It plays a vital role in maintaining the redox homeostasis due to the activation of the cellular antioxidant defense.

The glutamate-cystine antiporter mediates the exchange of extracellular L-cystine, the oxidized form of cysteine, and intracellular L-glutamate. The extracellularly moved glutamate is subjected to the action of EAAK. *Via* the uptake of cysteine, the system x_c^- has a central place in providing cysteine, the rate-limiting and critical precursor for glutathione biosynthesis in the cytosol, which is a major endogenous antioxidant and a key compound in maintaining the cellular redox balance. The system x_c^- has antioxidative protection, and also modulates diverse cellular processes, including the redox-dependent cell signaling.

The regulation of system x_c^- is complex. For example, an excess of extracellular glutamate blocks the cystine uptake (a competitive inhibitor for the x_c^- system) and depletes the cell cysteine. On the other hand, oxidative stress strongly induces the x_c^- system, as well as inflammatory stimuli.

There are also vesicular glutamate transporters (vGLUTs), a class (family) of three isoforms of intracellular transporters. They are the integral proteins of the synaptic vesicle membrane in neurons [15]. They mediate glutamate uptake from the cell cytosol into the synaptic vesicles. Out of two predominant isoforms, VGLUT1 and VGLUT2, VGLUT1 is mainly expressed in the cerebral and cerebellar cortices and hippocampus, whereas VGLUT2 is predominantly expressed in the diencephalon, brainstem, and spinal cord [16].

The dysregulation of glutamate transporters could contribute to brain pathologies or, to a lesser extent, be their primary cause [17]. Dysfunctional EAAT2/GLT-1, especially their down-regulation and/or alteration in their functions are often the initiating event or a part of the leading cascade of events in glutamate excitotoxicity and synaptic degeneration. According to a large number of studies, the detrimental effects of such dysregulation are implicated in the pathogenesis of various chronic and acute neurological disorders including Alzheimer's disease, Huntington's disease, amyotrophic lateral sclerosis, epilepsy, ischemia/stroke, traumatic brain injury, hepatic encephalopathy, brain tumors (malignant gliomas), as well as in human immunodeficiency virus 1-associated dementia and immune-mediated damage in multiple sclerosis. For the first time such findings were related to the brain ischemia and ALS. Moreover, the down-regulation of glutamate transporters (EAAT1 and EAAT2) is present in mental illnesses such as schizophrenia, depression, obsessive-compulsive disorders, autism and addiction [18]. These findings suggest that the modulation of EAAT2/GLT-1 may be of pharmacological interest. In fact, the activators of glutamate transporters and therapeutic up-regulation of their function and/or expression may be beneficial in a variety of pathological conditions in the brain. They could serve as potential treatment options because no therapies currently exist to modulate the glutamate transporters, although a number of substances have been explored for such purposes and the obtained results could be promising.

The Glutamate (GABA)-Glutamine Cycle

The compartmentation of glutamate and glutamine in neurons and glial cells is termed the glutamine-glutamate (GABA) cycle. In the metabolic pathway, this implies the release of glutamate or GABA from neurons into extracellular space (synaptic cleft), which are then taken up primarily into astrocytes, the cells extensively involved in the glutamine-glutamate cycle. They recycle glutamate *via* the glutamate-glutamine cycle and, together with glutamate derived from glycolysis in neuronal tissue (substantially smaller amounts), replenish the neuronal glutamate that was released after neuronal depolarization. The glutamate and GABA in astrocytes are converted into glutamine, or they are directed into the Krebs cycle located in the mitochondria. Glutamine is the most abundant amino acid and is the key compound in the glutamine-glutamate (GABA) cycle. Glutamine is

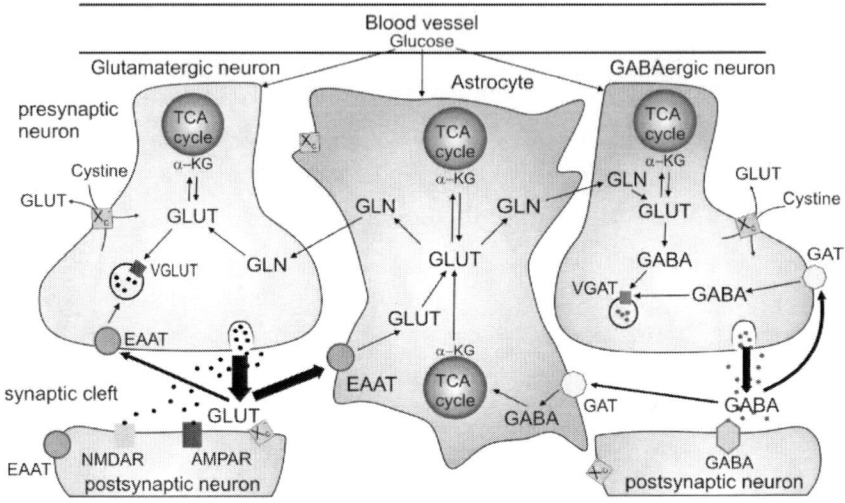

Figure 1. The glutamate (GABA)-glutamine cycle. The essential interactions between neurons (glutamatergic and GABAergic) and astrocytes. The release and uptake of neurotransmitters glutamate and GABA. The complex metabolic processes between glutamate (GLUT), GABA and glutamine (GLN). Abbreviations: α-KG: α-ketoglutarate; AMPAR: AMPA receptors; NMDAR: NMDA receptors; EAAT: excitatory amino acid transporter; GAT: GABA transporter; TCA cycle: tricarboxylic acid cycle; Xc$^-$: glutamate-cystine antiporter; VGAT: vesicular GABA transporter; VGLUT: vesicular glutamate transporter.

released from astrocytes into the extracellular space from where it will be taken up into GABAergic and glutamatergic neurons for usage, as a glutamate precursor and glutamate can serve as a source of GABA. Both of the synthesized neurotransmitters are then stored into vesicles as a pool from which they are released upon nerve terminal depolarization and the process continues to circle (Figure 1). The glutamine-glutamate (GABA) cycle, coupled with the consumption of a large part of the total brain energy demand, is the fundamental pathway for the regulation of concentration of these neurotransmitters. In addition to glutamate and GABA transporters, there are also membrane glutamine transporters that maintain its homeostasis.

All these complex activities provide, among others, the histological organization of the central nervous system cells. Astrocytes, which constitute the majority of glial cells within the brain and spinal cord, are located between blood vessels and neurons. They have intimate physical connections with synapses and blood vessels. Indeed, neurons and synapses are closely surrounded by glial cells and their processes. In that way the astrocytes are dynamically involved in modulating the complex neuronal functions and signaling, which generate and propagate electrical and chemical signals.

GLUTAMATE TRANSPORTERS: TARGETS FOR SCREENING EXOGENOUS REGULATORS AND OPPORTUNITIES FOR DEVELOPING NOVEL PHARMACOTHERAPEUTICS

The existent therapy for glutamate-mediated excitotoxity is insufficient, which also means that pharmacotherapy is insufficient for treating neurodegenerative and other diseases of the central nervous system apart from antagonists of glutamate receptors and compounds that target calcium influx. However, since the discovery of GLT-1/EAAT2 dynamic role in physiological, as well as in pathophysiological processes in the brain, the modulation of their expression and/or function has become a new therapeutic target in the aim to maintain the extracellular glutamate below neurotoxic levels in order to alleviate the glutamate-evoked cellular damage and neurologic deficits. These observations have prompted the searches for compounds that may modulate glutamate transporters. A tight regulation of glutamate transmission becomes a major pharmacological challenge in order to prevent and treat diseases in which the primary contributor might be the GLT-1/EAAT2 dysfunction. That's why a number of substances for transporter expression/activity improvement have been explored for decades as a neuroprotective drug target. Some of them are currently emerging as novel therapeutics and are considered to be promising tools for the treatment of neurodegenerative diseases. The situation is similar concerning the pharmacology and drug discovery relevant to amino acid transporters.

Rothstein et al., who already demonstrated the importance of glutamate transporters in maintaining normal brain function, as well as their involvement in the pathogenesis of some neurodegenerative diseases, focused their research on finding substances that could modify the activity of these transporters. In order to do that, they performed a blind screening study of 1,040 Food and Drug Administration approved drugs and nutritional agents for their bioactivity toward glutamate transporters, aiming to identify the effective agents as a potential treatment option for neurodegenerative diseases. This research is especially important when considering that pharmaceuticals that modulate EAAT2 expression and activity were not known until then. In that study, β-lactam antibiotics, together with several other substances, were identified for the first time as being powerful stimulators of some glutamate transporters, each of which increased GLT-1 by two times et least [1]. However, the expression of other transporters was not affected at all or was changed only to some degree, much less than EAAT2, indicating the selectivity of ceftriaxone in terms of the type of glutamate transporters whose expression could be increased by ceftriaxone. According to this unique activity, β-lactam antibiotics could serve as potential therapeutic agents for diseases other than bacterial, which was the discovery that determined the direction of many further research studies.

BETA-LACTAM ANTIBIOTICS

β-lactam antibiotics are a huge class of diverse compounds. They exist in oral, parenteral, and inhaled pharmaceutical formulations for clinical application. They are grouped together upon a shared structural feature. This implies an essential four-member beta-lactam ring in their molecular structure. Beside common structure, they share the same mechanism of antibacterial action by interfering with bacterial cell wall. These agents express bactericidal activity as they inhibit bacterial biosynthesis and interrupt cell-wall formation. This is the result of covalent binding to essential penicillin-binding proteins (three to eight enzymes per species) in both Gram-negative and Gram-positive bacteria.

There are four major β-lactam subgroups: penicillins, cephalosporins, monobactams and carbapenems. The effects of β-lactam antibiotics can be roughly divided into:

- Microbial and
- Non-antimicrobial.

In clinical practice, β-lactam antibiotics are currently used only in terms of their antibacterial effects. In spite of many positive results, the usage of their non-antimicrobial properties still has no place in clinical practice.

Antimicrobial Effects of β-Lactam Antibiotics

Since the 1940s, β-lactam antibiotics have been used to treat bacterial infections, due to the fact that penicillin, the ingredient responsible for antimicrobial effect, was isolated, and benzylpenicillin was produced in sufficient quantity for clinical use. The treatment of infectious diseases and their prognoses entered the modern era with this discovery.

Penicillin was the first antibiotic discovered and it was a natural product from the mold *Penicillium notatum*. This breakthrough in medicine was made by Alexander Fleming in 1928. The first generation of β-lactam antibiotics was followed by the discovery of the cephalosporins, and later by carbapenems and monocyclic β-lactams.

The spectrum of antibacterial activity varies within each class of the penicillin family. Each new class of β-lactam was developed to increase the antimicrobial coverage, either to increase the spectrum of activity and to include additional bacterial species, or to address specific resistance mechanisms that have arisen in the targeted bacterial population. Depending on the range of bacterial species susceptible to these agents, their activity was found to be efficient against many Gram-positive, Gram-negative and anaerobic organisms. Based on the structure and generation, β-lactam antibiotics belong either to the narrow, intermediate or broad spectrum antibacterials. They are well tolerated, effective and widely prescribed.

However, the reduction in antimicrobial effectiveness known for decades currently has a form of a global crisis. Bacterial resistance to antimicrobials, including β-lactam drugs, has become a reality. This problem is a matter of deep scientific concern both in hospital and outpatient settings. It is an inevitable consequence of the widespread inappropriate use of these drugs, both abuse and misuse in human medicine, agriculture and veterinary medicine. The greatest single cause of resistance to β-lactam antibiotics is bacterial synthesis (production) of one or several β-lactamases - a family of antibiotic-inactivating enzymes produced by bacteria, including anaerobes, which catalyze the hydrolysis of β-lactams, open the beta-lactam ring and generate the inactive β-lactam antibiotics. Inhibitors of β-lactamase have been developed in order to conserve the activity and extend the spectrum of β-lactam drugs against β-lactamase-producing organisms. The β-lactamase inhibitors (clavulanic acid, sulbactam and tazobactam) themselves have little direct antimicrobial activity, but when combined with an antibiotic they increase antibiotic stability against β-lactamases and extend their spectrum of activity.

Non-Antimicrobial Effects of β-Lactam Antibiotics

In addition to the antimicrobial properties, β-lactam antibiotic-triggered toxicity is well documented. Some of these drugs could have neurotoxic, nephrotoxic, gastrotoxic, hematotoxic or genotoxic effects. Moreover, some other organs and organic systems may be affected, too. These effects are designated as adverse drug reactions.

β-lactam antibiotics show capabilities that exceed their antimicrobial properties, due to which their use could be expected to increase in the future. Rothstein et al. gave the first proof of the non-antimicrobial effects of some substances out of 1,040 medications and other substances currently used in clinical practice. Overall, they tested all these substances *in vitro* (spinal cord slices and neurons, human astrocytes, as well as cell model of human diseases), and *in vivo* in rats and mice [1]. Some of the tested substances/drugs achieved the up-regulation of GLT-1 and modulation of their activity both *in vitro* and *in vivo*. These and several other research studies conducted *in vivo* - in mice and rats, including some models of glutamate neurotoxicity, as well as *in vitro* - on rodent and human fetal astrocytes, beside other cell lines and tissues, have shown that β-lactam antibiotics, which differ in molecular structure and pharmacokinetics, exhibit a large number of effects apart from antimicrobial, neuroprotective being the most prominent ones.

Rothstein et al. found that β-lactam antibiotics "increased both brain expression of GLT-1 and its biochemical and functional activity" [1]. Until this discovery, no substances were known to modulate the expression and activity of GLT-1/EAAT2. These concentration-dependent effects were exhibited by fifteen beta-lactam antibiotics in some rodent and human cell lines. Furthermore, ceftriaxone induced the up-regulation of GLT-1 in the hippocampus and spinal cord *in vivo*, as well in different cell lines. Other transporters were not affected at all or only to some degree, but much less than EAAT2, which was increased three times in comparison to the non-treated animals. However, other classes of antibiotics did not demonstrate the EAAT up-regulation, which indicates this activity to be selective since antimicrobial agents lacking a beta-lactam ring did not demonstrate such effects.

The next very important discovery of of Rothstein et al. study, that was registered for the very first time, was the neuroprotective effects of the identified up-regulation of GLT-1 evoked by β-lactam antibiotics [1]. The ceftriaxone induced up-regulation of GLT-1 was mediated by the increased transcription of the *EAAT2* gene which precedes the increase of GLT-1 expression. Nuclear factor-κB (NF-κB), expressed in neurons and glia, was found to be a regulator of this gene expression according to the results of Lee et al. who detected that the elevation of *EAAT2* transcription in primary fetal human astrocytes was NF-κB-mediated [19].

After the discovery of Rothstein et al., most further data concerning the non-antibacterial effects of β-lactam antibiotics refer to neuroprotection.

They were registered *in vitro* and *in vivo*. In the vast majority of research studies, a single β-lactam representative was observed. A particular emphasis was placed on ceftriaxone. Indeed, in preclinical but also in clinical settings, *in vitro* and in animal models of different neurological diseases, multiple neuroprotective effects were registered usually under the ceftriaxone treatment. For these reasons, it would not be reliable to conclude that all beta-lactams, apart from ceftriaxone, possess such a wide range of neuroprotective effects, and the positive effects of ceftriaxone cannot automatically be ascribed to them.

Due to the multiple non-antimicrobial mechanisms of action, although the central site appears to have an increased expression of GLT-1 mRNA levels, the protective effects of beta lactam antibiotics, ceftriaxone in the first place, were reported in various experimental models of human neurological diseases. These are, for example, ALS, stroke, epileptic seizures, Alzheimer's, Huntington's, Parkinson's disease, multiple sclerosis and other neurological diseases, traumatic brain injury, HIV-associated neurocognitive disorder, some psychiatric illnesses, suppression of various types of pain, the treatment of substance use disorders, addiction and tolerance (cocaine, alcohol, nicotine, morphine, etc.) [20].

CEFTRIAXONE

In the last fifteen years, since the discovery of Rothstein et al. concerning the neurological effects of ceftriaxone, this antimicrobial has become very attractive to the entire scientific community. Since then it has been investigated whether it can be disease-modifying in many neurological and psychiatric disorders and diseases [21].

Like penicillin, the naturally occurring penicillinase-stable, cephalosporin C, a cephalosporin antibiotic, was also discovered by accident by an Italian scientist Giuseppe Brotzu in 1945. He originally derived it from an extract from the fungus *Acremonium chrysogenum*, previously known as *Cephalosporium acremonium*, which could produce at least five different antibiotics. The extract isolated from this mold demonstrated antimicrobial activity against both Gram-positive and Gram-negative bacteria. However, the structure of the cephalosporin C was elucidated in 1959, and this antimicrobial class achieved clinical utility in the 1960s since the first cephalosporin was sold in 1964. Thereafter plenty of novel cephalosporins were developed. Today, cephalosporins account for nearly half of the prescriptions out of all β-lactams.

The cephalosporin family consists of five generations. They exist in pharmaceutical formulations for oral and parenteral applications. The first generation of cephalosporins is efficient predominantly against Gram-positive bacteria. The successive generations got a broader spectrum of activity: an increased activity against Gram-negative bacteria and a greater resistance to beta-lactamases, i.e., there is a generational shift from Gram-positive to Gram-negative coverage and resistance to β-lactamases. This became clear with the third generation of cephalosporins.

Ceftriaxone belongs to the third-generation of cephalosporin antibiotics. It efficiently penetrates the blood-brain barrier. It demonstrates strong neuroprotective effects in various models of both *in vitro* and *in vivo* models of glutamate central nervous system neurotoxicity due to its multifaceted activity. At first, it increases the glutamate reuptake by up-regulating GLT-1 expression. It stimulates EAAT2 expression in human and rat astrocytes, rodent cultured spinal cord slices, as well as *in vivo*. It has no effect on EAAT1 and GLAST expression [1, 19].

According to the study of Rothstein et al., in healthy rats, ceftriaxone was given daily for 5-7 days at a dose of 200 mg/kg body weight intraperitoneally [1]. The up-regulation of GLT-1 was registered within 48 hours after initial treatment. There was a triple increase in the expression of GLT protein in the hippocampus and spinal cord. These effects lasted for three months. There was also an increase in GLT-1-mediated glutamate transport (ceftriaxone biochemical effects). The increased GLT-1 expression was mediated *via* transcription of the *GLT1* gene, indicating the genetic level of ceftriaxone action. Consequently, the effects of ceftriaxone are expected to be neuroprotective.

Beside glutamatergic regulation, the non-antimicrobial activity of ceftriaxone leads to neuroprotection due to the large number of other mechanisms. These are especially numerous in the field of oxidative stress and antioxidant defense. For example, a free radical scavenging property of ceftriaxone has been observed. Due to the interaction with transition metal (II) ions, it exhibits metal chelating properties [22]. Furthermore, increased activities of antioxidant enzymes SOD, catalase, glutathione reductase and glutathione peroxidase, together with simultaneous decrement of lipid peroxidation, were registered in different brain pathologies of rats treated with ceftriaxone [23]. Overall, the reduction of oxidative stress by ceftriaxone and the demonstration of its antioxidant action have been well established.

Moreover, anti-inflammatory effects of ceftriaxone were documented at least in traumatic brain injury where it reduced pro-inflammatory cytokines interleukin-1 [beta], interferon-[gamma], and tumor necrosis factor-[alpha] [24]. Apart from these anti-inflammatory effects, its immunomodulatory activity was found, too.

Thus, ceftriaxone provides neuroprotective potential *via* anti-excitotoxic, anti-inflammatory, and antioxidant activities. Ceftriaxone is found to:

- demonstrate an increased expression and activity of GLT-1, through an increased transcription of the *EAAT2* gene,
- regulate cystine/glutamate transporter (SLC7A11). Lewerenz et al. concluded: "Ceftriaxone acts as an inducer of system x_c^- in glial and neuronal cells (cortical and spinal) … independently of its effect on excitatory amino acid transporters by induction of the transcription factor Nrf2 (nuclear factor erythroid 2-related factor 2), a known inducer of system x(c)(-), and the specific x(c)(-) subunit xCT" [25],
- possess free radical scavenging and metal chelating properties,
- possess anti-inflammatory and immunomodulatory properties,
- bind to α-synuclein and inhibit its polymerization [26],
- modulate expression of genes related to β-amyloid metabolism and ameliorate tau pathology [27].

The unique ceftriaxone function is predominantly based on the increase in GLT-1 in the rat brain, which modulates the transport of glutamate, placing it in potential neurotherapeutics. Accordingly, it may be able to manage specific neurodegenerative disorders where the excessive extracellular glutamate is at least a part of their pathogenesis. This result could be achieved with the "doses routinely used for treating infections of the central nervous system", and with concentrations of ceftriaxone in the central nervous system comparable to the levels that exist in the treatment of meningitis [1].

Ceftriaxone in the Prevention and Treatment of Diseases Related to Glutamate Excitotoxicity

Neurodegenerative diseases are characterized by a progressive loss of neuronal structure and function in selective vulnerable central nervous system regions. It is believed that neurodegeneration and a great number of neurological disorders are at least partly dependent on the excessive receptor stimulation with glutamate that could, beside other reasons, be also due to the reduction of GLT-1 expression. The so-called excitotoxic neurologic and mental diseases already mentioned above, impair patient's health, sometimes to the devastating level, and represent a significant economic burden to the individual and society as a whole. So, any substance that could modify these diseases is very welcome, especially in the case of neurodegenerative diseases for which currently available drugs are not disease-modifying. The most positive results currently exist for ceftriaxone. It has already been successfully and extensively studied preclinically in prevention and/or treatment of a number of such diseases. However, a great efficacy obtained in preclinical studies (*in vitro* and in experimental animals) cannot be accurately transferred to clinical trials in humans for many reasons. Thus, the substances/drugs leading to the regulation of GLT-1 expression/function/biochemistry, including ceftriaxone, are still far from clinical practice even though they represent significant advances in this field of pharmacology.

The Effects of Ceftriaxone in Neurodegenerative Disorders

Amyotrophic Lateral Sclerosis

Amyotrophic lateral sclerosis (ALS) is a rare, multifactorial, late-onset, rapid and fatal neuromuscular disorder with median survival time of 3-5 years. It was first described by Jean-Martin Charcot in the 1870s. The progressive degeneration of upper and lower motor neurons and surrounding glial cells leads to the voluntary muscle weakness and death usually due to respiratory failure.

In most cases ALS is sporadic. About 10% of patients have familial (inherited) autosomal dominant fashion. Genetic cause was also identified in 10% of patients without a known family history. Mutations in gene for the enzyme copper/zinc superoxide dismutase 1 (SOD1) is found in 10-20% of familial ALS. This was the first ALS mutation, discovered in 1993.

The most prominent findings in ALS were those of Rothstein et al. [1, 17]. In postmortem brains of ALS sufferers they registered "selective loss of glial glutamate transporter GLT-1, but not of GLAST and EAAT1", especially in motor cortex and spinal cord, pointing at a relevant role of these proteins in the pathogenesis of ALS in humans [17]. The findings in mutant mouse models of this disease were similar. Namely, the focal loss of the astroglial EAAT2 in the spinal cord of rats appears very early and precedes neuronal degeneration and motor neuron death. Besides an enormous loss of glutamate transporters and glutamate excitotoxicity, mitochondrial dysfunction, oxidative stress, inflammation, etc. were also found in ALS.

Despite intensive research, pharmacotherapy of ALS is still extremely discouraging. By targeting known pathophysiological pathways toward a glial glutamate transporter, a number of experimental research, preclinical and ALS clinical trials have been done aiming to determine which effects could be achieved by the application of ceftriaxone. In the study conducted by Rothstein et al., cephalosporin antibiotics were the only class of compounds active in the majority of ALS-related assays [1]. The beneficial effects of ceftriaxone were registered in the mutant superoxide dismutase 1 transgenic mice ALS model, in terms of slowing the progression of the disease and prolonging muscular stability. In their conclusion Rothstein et al. stated that "the drug delayed the loss of neurons, increased muscle strength, moderately increased the life span and increased mouse survival". However, the connection between ceftriaxone use for any antibacterial reason and improvement in ALS in humans was registered accidentally much earlier, in 1994, but the results were not uniform and satisfactory, so the testing of ceftriaxone in ALS was abandoned [28].

Out of all the diseases in which ceftriaxone could be applied therapeutically, only the studies in ALS patients reached the level of clinical trial which was conducted in the period between Sept 4th, 2006 and July 30th, 2012 [29]. This randomized, double-blind, placebo-controlled, multicenter trial involved 66 patients divided into three groups. The first group received daily intravenously 2 grams of ceftriaxone, the second one 4 grams divided into two doses, and the third one was given a placebo. This was a three-stage clinical study. The first stage lasted for seven days and was conducted in order to determine ceftriaxone pharmacokinetics. In the second stage which lasted for 20 weeks, the pre-specified criteria for safety and tolerability were studied, while in the third one the primary endpoints pre-specified for the efficacy on disease progression were monitored (survival and functional decline). Both doses of ceftriaxone were well tolerated and achieved the target cerebrospinal fluid concentrations. Stage 3 included 66 participants from stages 1 and 2 and 448 new participants (n = 554). In stages one and two, the functional decline was slower in ceftriaxone 4g-treated group, compared to placebo. However, such success was not registered in stage three, in which the survival differences between groups were not found. Adverse events, sometimes intolerable, were more common in the ceftriaxone than in the placebo group. The authors of this trial concluded: "Despite promising stage 2 data, stage 3 of this trial of ceftriaxone in amyotrophic lateral sclerosis did not show clinical efficacy". This clinical trial has been recently finalized. The promising protective effects of ceftriaxone obtained in ALS animal models were absent in ALS sufferers and preclinical beneficial effects of ceftriaxone did not translate into clinical conditions. However, this research has made some progress in the approach to ALS, and the results obtained require an extremely studious analysis.

Alzheimer's Disease

Originally described by Alois Alzheimer in 1907, Alzheimer's disease (AD), a progressive age-related neurodegenerative disorder, is the most common type of dementia in the elderly. It affects 6-8% of the population aged 65 and 30% of the population aged 85. Together with other types of dementia, AD is the fourth leading cause of mortality and morbidity worldwide. In spite of multiple hypotheses of ethiopathogenesis, the exact and primary mechanism of AD is still unknown. It remains that AD is a very complex interplay between many internal and external factors and processes in its occurrence and development. The terminal effects are the loss of synapses and neuronal death, neurochemical and pathological changes.

The disruption in glutamatergic signaling has been reported in both animal models of AD and people with dementia. Beside glutamate excitotoxicity, GLT-1/EAAT2 dysfunction (significant reduction or damage) is found in AD. Jacob et al. found the "impairment in the expression of excitatory amino acid transporters (EAAT1 and EAAT2) at both gene and protein levels in hippocampus and gyrus frontalis medialis of AD patients, already in the early clinical stages of the disease. The loss of EAAT immunoreactivity was particularly obvious in the vicinity of amyloid plaques" [30]. The reduced function of glutamate transportation was found to be associated with a decreased EAAT2 protein expression in AD brains. Such impairments were accompanied by Aβ-related neuropathology and *vice versa*: Aβ1–42 induces GLT-1/EAAT2 internalization in astrocytes, thereby losing their regulatory function in glutamate homeostasis [31]. Furthermore, the reduced GLT-1/EAAT2 was registered in cognitive impairment. However, the sequence of GLT-1/EAAT2 - Aβ-related events has not been clarified yet.

In different animal models of AD, the application of ceftriaxone was successful in suppressing genetic, protein and behavioral damage [21]. The most prominent effects were the significant regulation of GLT-1 expression, as well as N-glutamine transporter 1, particularly pronounced around the amyloid plaque. A reduction of tau accumulation was also observed [27].

Tikhonova et al. registered an increased density of pyramidal neurons in CA1 region of hippocampus of rats indicating a stimulation of neurogenesis by ceftriaxon [21]. The improvement of damaged cognitive and movement functions were also achieved. Furthermore, strong genetic changes evoked by ceftriaxone were determined which were directed towards the defense against factors involved in many AD processes. For example, ceftriaxone induced the down-regulation of Bace1 (encoding β-secretase BACE1 involved in Aβ production) and Ace2 (encoding enzymes involved in Aβ degradation) mRNA levels in the hypothalamus, as well as some genes that encode enzymes involved in Aβ degradation [32, 27].

In a number of studies ceftriaxone was effective against oxidative disbalance in the applied models of AD, which is of great importance when considering the fact that impaired calcium homeostasis and the excessive accumulation of ROS in AD patients may induce mitochondrial dysfunction, increased production and aggregation of Aβ and promotion of the phosphorylation of tau protein [33]. Oxidative stress is among the most exploited and most documented disturbances in AD although the exact mechanisms underlying the disruption of redox balance still remain unresolved.

Having in mind the cholinergic hypothesis of AD and a cholinergic deficit and increased levels of acetylcholine as one of the hallmarks of AD, improvements achieved by ceftriaxone result from the fact that it attenuates the cholinergic disturbances [33].

The aluminum hypothesis of AD ethiopathogenesis is more than half a century old. During this period, biochemical and structural changes in the brain and neurobehavioral alterations have remained the same or resembled those found in AD. The basic pathophysiological characteristics of AD - the aggregation of beta-amyloid peptide into the amyloidal plaques placed extracellularly or in the walls of cerebral blood vessels, and neurofibrillary tangles in the neurons and glial cells, were among those changes [34]. Aluminum has also been found in senile plaques in post-mortem human brains of AD patients. Moreover, in aluminum neurotoxicity, similar to those in AD pathology, a cholinergic deficit, a disorder of mitochondrial function and glucose metabolism, oxidative stress, neuroinflammation, a dysfunction in neurotransmission and cell signaling, etc. were registered [34, 35, 36]. Poor performance in cognitive tests was registered in workers occupationally exposed to aluminum, but also in acute aluminum exposed rats [37]. Exposure to aluminum can lead to neuronal and astroglial damage and death in susceptible brain regions. The evidence that aluminum causes AD is still inconclusive and a matter of scientific interest. However, so far there have been no studies investigating whether ceftriaxone could change aluminum neurotoxic effects, which is the topic of this chapter.

Convulsions and Epilepsy

Epilepsy is a severe and chronic group of associated neurodegenerative diseases. It affects all age groups, can significantly impair quality of life and has substantial both direct and indirect costs. It is characterised by periodic occurrence of spontaneous convulsive or nonconvulsive seizures as the consequence of abnormal hypersynchronus electrical activity caused by an imbalance between neuronal excitatory and inhibitory (glutamate-GABA) transmitter activities, with dominance of the hyperexcitability. Astrocytes have a crucial role in protecting neurons from hyperexcitability and a certain role of GLT-1 in the epileptogenesis has been established in several studies in animals and humans. Although these findings are not completely consistent, the predominant evidence shows an increased animal susceptibility to convulsions if astrocytic glutamate transporters are reduced or completely missing. This is consistent with the findings of Tanaka et al. concerning lethal spontaneous seizure appearance and premature death in homozygous mice deficient in GLT-1 (global deletion of GLT-1, first showed that a deficit in EAAT2 caused neurological problems in mice) and those of Petr et al. concerning the deletion of astrocytic GLT-1, but not neuronal, as well as its correlation with spontaneus seizures [38, 39]. However, the impact of the regional GLT-1 distribution and incomplete deletion of GLT-1 on spontaneous lethal and nonlethal convulsions has to be investigated [40]. There is also evidence of decreased glutamate transporter expressions (EAAT1 and EAAT2) in cortical dysplastic tissues of patients operated for medically intractable epilepsy [41].

The evidence about GLT-1 involvement in the pathogenesis of epilepsy indicates that an enhancing GLT-1/EAAT2 expression could be a potential therapeutic approach in treating convulsions [42]. Thus, ceftriaxone, an agent that increases the expression of EAT/GLT-1, could represent a new neuroprotective agent especially due to the presence of therapeutic failure in 30% of patients. Because of these capabilities, ceftriaxone was applied in various convulsive experimental models produced by chemical or electrical stimuli. In the pentylenetetrazole (PTZ, a GABA antagonist) kindling, ceftriaxone (200 mg/kg/12hrs ip, during three consecutive days) exhibited anticonvulsant effects. It increased the latency to the convulsion onset and decreased seizure duration [43]. Also, markers of oxidative stress evoked by PTZ were attenuated with ceftriaxone pretreatment. Zeng et al. demonstrated the involvement of astrocytes in the pathogenesis of epilepsy and „decreased extracellular glutamate levels, neuronal death, seizure frequency, and improved survival" with ceftiaxone in tuberous sclerosis complex [44]. In a study of two strains of mice pre-treated with ceftriaxone (200mg/kg ip, during five consecutive days), the protective effects in PTZ-induced convulsions were related to the frequency and latency of generalized clonic seizure, generalized tonic-clonic seizure, and convulsion-associated deaths [45]. In addition to clinical findings, Uyanikgil et al. recorded anticonvulsive effects of ceftriaxone electroencephalografically [46]. Having in mind the basic non-antimicrobial effect of ceftriaxone, all the above mentioned studies indicate that astrocytic glutamate uptake protects neurons from hyperexcitability.

Even though considered to be generally safe, the proconvulsant activity of beta-lactam antibiotics has been reported in humans. The first convulsive episode of penicillin administered intrathecally was registered in 1947. So far, many convulsive seizures have been reported as an adverse effect of beta lactam antibiotics. Moreover, acute neurotoxic effects of penicillin and some other beta lactams, applied in certain appropriate doses, could induce hyperexcitability and could have epileptogenic potential in experimental animals. Thus, they are used in various animal species to establish different experimental patterns of epileptic seizures. Such models are very useful for the investigation of epilepsy pathogenesis and anticonvulsant substances.

All in all, based on literature data, beta-lactam antibiotics could have quite opposite effects in relation to convulsions. However, proconvulsant and anticonvulsant effects do not exclude each other because the activity of these drugs on the neuronal excitability seems to depend not only on their type, but also on the dose, way and duration of their administration. Therefore, the relationship between beta-lactam antibiotics and epilepsy is required to be studied further on.

POSSIBLE THERAPEUTIC EFFECTS OF CEFTRIAXONE AGAINST ALUMINUM NEUROTOXICITY APPLIED BEFORE AND AFTER ALUMINUM

Aluminum, although a nonessential element in the human body, has been found to alter various metabolic reactions and cause deleterious effects in human health. Beside in humans, its effects are investigated in a wide variety of studies performed both *in vitro* and *in vivo*. However, the most thoroughly examined and documented are its pro-oxidant effects and consequently developed oxidative stress. During these processes, the mechanisms of antioxidant protection could be spent or even exhausted. The terminal outcome is the oxidative damage of proteins, lipids, and DNA and the dysfunction and damage of biological membranes. This is likely to be one of the mechanisms of aluminum neurotoxicity.

Bearing in mind numerous aluminum neurotoxic effects in humans and in experiments of different designs, there is a need for an agent that could prevent or treat these effects. Since the glutamate excitotoxicity is in the basis of aluminum toxicity, the GLT-1/EAAT2 targeting *via* ceftriaxone may be neuroprotective in the case of this neurotoxicity.

Materials and Methods

Animals and Experimental Design

Male adult Wistar rats, 12 weeks old at the beginning of the experiments, were used for this study, 9-12 animals for each group. The animals were provided with commercial food and water *ad libitum,* and were housed in transparent Plexiglas cages under a 12h/12h light/dark cycle at a temperature of 23 ± 2°C. The research protocol was approved by the local Ethics Committee for animal experimentation and was strictly in accordance with the "Guidelines for Animal Study No 282–12/2002" (Military Medical Academy, Belgrade, Serbia), which is in harmony with international regulations.

After being intraperitoneally anesthetized with sodium thiopental (Specia, Paris) (0.04 g/kg body weight), rats were placed on a stereotaxic instrument for small animals and *via* stereotaxic brain surgery the examined substances (saline, aluminum chloride) were administered through a Hamilton micro syringe into the left brain hemisphere Cornu Ammonis region 1 (CA1) of hippocampus. The position for the injection was determined relative to the lambda suture, defined from its center: 3.1 mm dorsally, 4.3 mm laterally and 2.5 mm ventrally from the skull surface [47]. According to the design of the research, ceftriaxone was applied intraperitoneally.

The recovery period after the brain treatment lasted for 12 days. Each rat was kept in a separate cage during that time. Thereafter they were sacrificed by decapitation. The heads were flash-frozen in liquid nitrogen and stored at -70 °C until brain samples were prepared for biochemical analysis.

Treatments

The rats were randomly assigned to treatments. Based on the applied substances, they were divided into four groups: the first group received a single dose of 0.9 per cent w/v NaCl (NaCl, control group), the second one a single dose of aluminum chloride (Sigma-Aldrich, USA) in a dose of 3.7×10^{-4} g/kg body weight dissolved in sterile deionized water (AlCl3, aluminum group). Both substances were applied intrahippocampally in the volume of 0.01 ml. The rats in the third and fourth group were intraperitoneally treated with ceftriaxone (Azaren, Panfarma, Vršac, Serbia) in a daily dose of 200 mg/kg body weight. It was administered during five consecutive days before (Cef+AlCl3, third group) and after the single dose of aluminum chloride (AlCl3+Cef, fourth group), i.e., the first dose of ceftriaxone in the fourth group was given immediately after the aluminum treatment. Ceftriaxone was applied in the volume of 2 ml/kg body weight. The first two groups received saline intraperitoneally in the same volume as ceftriaxone.

Assay of Biochemical Analyses in Brain Tissues

The analyses of biochemical parameters were performed in crude mitochondrial fractions from the brain regions ipsilateral to the injection site. They were determined in five brain regions: the forebrain cortex (FbC), basal forebrain (BFb), striatum (S), hippocampus (H) and cerebellum (Cereb). Brains were kept on ice while being dissected.

The activity of glucose-6-phosphate dehydrogenase (G6PDH, EC 1.1.1.49) and cytochrome c oxydase (Complex IV, EC 1.9.3.1) was determined by the methods of Bergmeyer, and Hess and Pope, respectively [48, 49]. The content of reduced glutathione (GSH) was determined by the method of Anderson [50]. The GSH abbreviation is used to designate the reduced form of glutathione.

Statistical Analysis

Data were expressed as means ± SD. The Student's t-test was used for comparisons between groups. Statistical significance was determined at probability level of $p < 0.05$.

Results and Discussion

Neurotoxic Effects of Aluminum

The exposure to aluminum can induce several biological disturbances. Although being a non-redox metal, it can act as a pro-oxidant. In the results displayed, the intrahippocampal application of aluminum chloride caused changes of all the examined biochemical analyses. They were not registered only at the injection site, i.e., in the CA1 sector of the hippocampus, but also in other parts of the brain, indicating extensive spatial spreading of the damage, as the result of regional differences in neuronal and metabolic pathways, including neurotransmitters, but also in different brain neuronal circuits [51, 52, 53]. The decline of tested parameters was found in the forebrain cortex, striatum, basal forebrain, hippocampus and cerebellum, some of which are selectively vulnerable in AD pathology (hippocampus, forebrain cortex) (Figures 2, 3, 4). The hierarchy of the brain structures susceptibility to aluminum toxicity is similar to the one seen in AD. These results are in agreement with other findings that had shown the inhibitory effects of aluminum against several antioxidant enzymes in different parts of the brain, as well as its pro-oxidant effects [4, 34, 35, 36, 54]. It was evident that aluminum exhibited its toxic effects in both the cytosol and mitochondria.

The activity of *glucose-6-phosphate dehydrogenase* was dramatically decreased in all structures. In comparison to the control group, the significance of $p < 0.01$ was observed in all brain structures of aluminum-treated animals (Figure 2). This shows that one of the harmful targets in aluminum toxicity is hexose monophosphate shunt (the oxidative pentose phosphate pathway, PPP), demonstrated by measuring the activity of G6PDH, the first and rate limiting enzyme in this pathway. This is a metabolic pathway that runs entirely in the cytosol. One of the PPP major functions in this process of glucose degradation is to produce (regenerate) the reducing agent NADPH from its oxidized form NADP+, which is, beside in cytosol, also produced in mitochondria. The PPP is the predominant source of NADPH, a key compound in preserving the oxidative-reductive balance and suppressing the effects of excessive production of free radicals and oxidative stress. In order to achieve the PPP function, the GPDH enzyme activity must be preserved, which is dramatically damaged by aluminum. This makes conditions for an inadequate defense against free radical production whose inevitable consequence is oxidative stress. Thus, the

GPDH enzyme supplementation could suppress aluminum neurotoxicity [55].

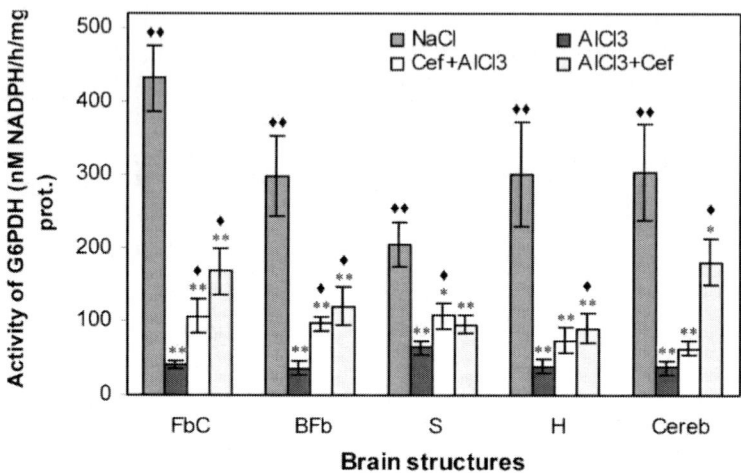

Figure 2. The activity of glucose-6-phosphate dehydrogenase in the brain of Wistar rats (n = 9–12), intra-hippocampally treated with 0.9% NaCl and aluminum chloride ($AlCl_3$) and with ceftriaxone (200mg/kg body weight, intraperitoneally, during five consecutive days) before (Cef+$AlCl_3$ group) and after aluminum chloride application ($AlCl_3$+Cef group). The values were expressed as mean ± SD. $p < 0.05$, $p < 0.01$ are the levels of statistical significance found versus 0.9% NaCl (*, **) and versus $AlCl_3$-treated rats (♦, ♦♦) (Student's t-test). The rats were sacrificed 12 days after intra-hippocampal treatments.

Cytochrome c oxydase (Complex IV) is an enzyme that belongs to the respiratory electron transport chain of oxidative phosphorylation located into mitochondria. By affecting the iron homeostasis, aluminum acts detrimentally to the respiratory chain enzymes. The strongest reduction of Complex IV was registered in the hippocampus, forebrain cortex and cerebellum ($p < 0.01$), compared to the control, and the other two structures were also affected (striatum, basal forebrain) ($p < 0.05$) (Figure 3). This respiratory chain includes four large protein complexes (I–IV), and ATP synthase (complex V) [56]. All of these subunits are embedded into the internal mitochondrial membrane. During the mitochondrial part of glycolysis, through which pyruvate is completely oxidized, the cellular energy molecule (ATP) is generated, much more than in glycolysis to the degree of pyruvate production, which occurs in the cytoplasm. The Complex IV, the last enzyme in the respiratory chain, which receives and transmits electrons, precedes ATP production which is deteriorated by the mitochondrial dysfunction [15].

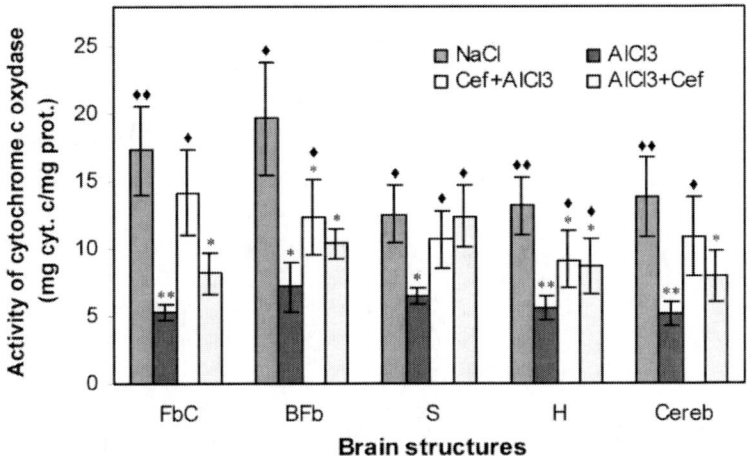

Figure 3. The activity of cytochrome c oxydase (Complex IV) in the brain of Wistar rats (n = 9–12) intra-hippocampally treated with 0.9% NaCl and aluminum chloride (AlCl$_3$), and with ceftriaxone (200mg/kg body weight, intraperitoneally, during five consecutive days) before (Cef+AlCl$_3$ group) and after aluminum chloride application (AlCl$_3$+Cef group). The values were expressed as mean ± SD. $p < 0.05$, $p < 0.01$ are the levels of statistical significance found versus 0.9% NaCl (*, **) and versus AlCl$_3$-treated rats (♦, ♦♦) (Student's t-test). The rats were sacrificed 12 days after intra-hippocampal treatments.

The impaired function of cytochrome c oxidase, which was induced by aluminum, must inevitably be accompanied by an increased production of free radicals since this enzyme is very strongly involved in the oxido-reductive reactions, due to the fact that mitochondria are the place of free radical production. "Being involved in the production of reactive oxygen species, aluminum may impair mitochondrial bioenergetics and may lead to the generation of oxidative stress" [34]. The occurrence of cellular oxidative stress due to mitochondrial dysfunction is one of proposed mechanisms responsible for neurodegenerative diseases.

The reduced glutathione (GSH) content was decreased in all brain structures of animals treated with aluminum ($p < 0.05$) in comparison to the saline treated rats (Figure 4). That could be caused by the increased oxidative stress and/or the decreased GSH synthesis/regeneration, especially in the neurons, which are more vulnerable to free radicals than glial cells due to multiple reasons. This most abundant non-protein thiol in cells represents the main compound in the regulation of cellular redox homeostasis (maintaining the intracellular redox balance) and is a part of overall cellular antioxidant defense system which has extremely high redox potential.

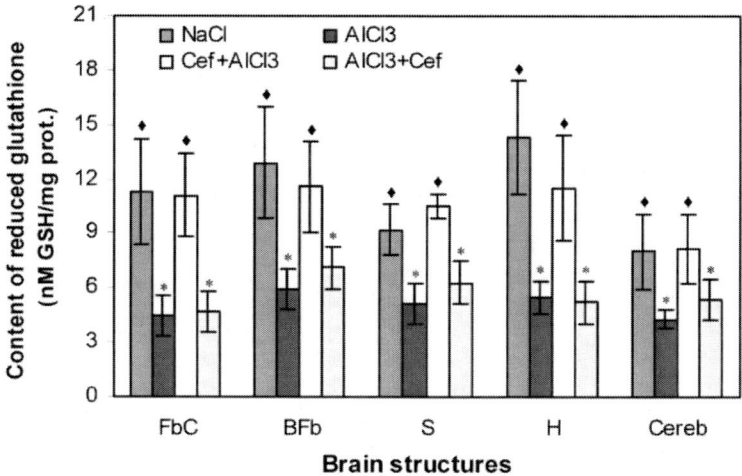

Figure 4. The content of reduced glutathione in the brain of Wistar rats (n = 9–12) intra-hippocampally treated with 0.9% NaCl and aluminum chloride ($AlCl_3$), and with ceftriaxone (200mg/kg body weight, intraperitoneally, during five consecutive days) before (Cef+$AlCl_3$ group) and after aluminum chloride application ($AlCl_3$+Cef group). The values were expressed as mean ± SD. $p < 0.05$, $p < 0.01$ are the levels of statistical significance found versus 0.9% NaCl (*, **) and versus $AlCl_3$-treated rats (♦, ♦♦) (Student's t-test). The rats were sacrificed 12 days after intra-hippocampal treatments.

Alterations in the pentose phosphate pathway and disruption of the mitochondrial glycolysis sequence, which in this study relates to complex IV, are very dangerous for cell functions. This can be quite reliable in the case of diminished level of reduced glutathione, which accounts for as much as 95% and more of total glutathione. It is reversibly oxidized to GSSH form in the processes of oxidative stress prevention and antioxidant defense. Astrocytes are the major source of glutathione in the brain, which are subjected to reactivation and apoptosis in the case of aluminum neurotoxicity [57].

The GSH-GSSG-GSH cycle and reduction of GSSH back to GSH is disrupted in the above stated conditions caused by aluminum. Such dysregulation of GSH contributes to the pathogenesis of many health disturbances since GSH is, beside being antioxidant, an ubiquitous cofactor for the glutathione dependent enzymes, it is involved in redox signaling, and it is vital in the detoxification of xenobiotics and/or their metabolites, in the regulation of cell proliferation, apoptosis, immune function, apoptosis and cell survival.

The Effects of Ceftriaxone on the Toxic Effects of Aluminum Chloride Given before and after the Application of Aluminum

In order to reverse the damaging effects of glutamate caused by aluminum toxicity, it was necessary to decrease its levels. In the case of a very high potential of aluminum neurotoxicity, the effect of ceftriaxone against aluminum neurotoxicity was, according to our knowledge, for the first time examined in this study. In general, it was demonstrated that ceftriaxone application was beneficial whether it was applied during standard procedure before the injection of aluminum into the hippocampus, or after it. The pre-treatment with ceftriaxone resulted in the improvement of all aluminum-induced detrimental effects concerning the analyzed biochemical parameters. In the case of enhanced oxidative stress induced by aluminum, as it was demonstrated by low activity of G6PDH and cytochrome c oxidase, and by low level of GSH, ceftriaxone prevented or ameliorated the development of these events (Figure 2, 3, 4).

A number of studies provided evidence that astrocytes, together with microglia, were involved in aluminum toxicity as aluminum accumulates in the mitochondria and astrocytes. In that way it disrupts some mitochondrial functions with a consequent energy reduction which could amplify the excitotoxic injury. Furthermore, the astrocytic accumulation of aluminum disrupts the astrocytic glutamate uptake, with secondary excitotoxicity and neuronal damage [58]. Beside other effects, high levels of glutamate reduce glutathione production intracellularly by inhibiting the cystine/glutamate antiporter. On the other hand, ceftriaxone has a quite opposite effect on this antiporter since it induces it [25]. This is one, but not the only way how ceftriaxone counteracts the toxic effects of aluminum.

Aluminum induced reactivity of astrogliosis contributes to the pathophysiology of neurodegenerative diseases, including AD [59]. In the injured brain cells, astroglial cells react by rapidly producing more glial fibrillary acidic protein (GFAP), a highly specific marker for astrocyte cells. The reactive astrogliosis is fundamental for the evolution and resolution of neuropathology [60].

The up-regulation of GFAP staining, indicating the increased expression of GFAP due to reactive astroglial changes as the response to neuronal damage and inflammation after intrahippocampally applied aluminum, was demonstrated to show the marked involvement of astroglia in aluminum neurotoxicity [61]. This is one of the possible mechanisms by which aluminum causes toxic effects in rat brain, with glutamate excitotoxicity as the most prominent effect. Therefore, it was not surprising that ceftriaxone, already known for the up-regulation of GLT, given during five consecutive days prior to aluminum, protected cells from aluminum excitotoxicity, determined by G6PDH and cytochrome c activity, and by the level of GSH. Moreover, the most powerful effects were shown at the GSH level, where the detrimental effect of aluminum was reverted to the control values ($p < 0.05$ in all brain structures). That was possible, at the first, because of a very strong interference of ceftriaxone with mitochondrial electron respiratory chain, which can be seen through the increased activity of cytochrome c oxidase in all the examined brain structures ($p < 0.05$). Consequently, the production of free radicals could be reduced, together with the increased synthesis of ATP, which all leads to a higher level of GSH. The reduced glutathione is synthesized in the cytosol of astrocytes and neurons, with higher levels found in astrocytes. It is predominantly localized in three compartments: cytosol (about 80%), mitochondria (about 10%) and the rest in endoplasmatic reticulum. GSH in the mitochondria is particularly important in defending both physiologically and pathologically generated oxidative stress in the mitochondrial respiration.

In addition to enhanced mitochondrial activity, the increased G6PDH activity contributed to an increase in the level of GSH. This enzyme is required for the production of the reducing equivalents (NADPH), which are necessary for the adequate function of oxidative phosphorylation and antioxidant defense. NADPH is, in fact, the essential supplier of reducing equivalents. Thus, the increased NADPH production, together with the improved production of ATP, is a prerequisite for the resynthesis of GSH. Indeed, GSSG can be reduced back to GSH at the expense of NADPH and ATP. The increased GPDH activity induced by pretreatment with ceftriaxone was registered in the forebrain cortex, basal forebrain and striatum ($p < 0.05$), but not in the hippocampus, the region directly damaged by aluminum, nor in cerebellum. So, the positive effects of ceftriaxone were the least pronounced in relation to G6PDH. But, together with other positive effects of ceftriaxone, they were still sufficient to bring about a complete recovery of the GSH. This could be additionally ascribed to metal chelating and free radical scavenging properties of ceftriaxone and the improved x_c^- system.

Indeed, the neuroprotective effects of ceftriaxone in aluminum neurotoxicity could be achieved due to its dual action: on the one hand, it affects GLT-1/EAAT2 expression/function, and, on the other hand, it diminishes the blocking of system x_c^- induced by the excess of the extracellular glutamate. In the later case, the up-regulation of glutamate/cystine transporter system x_c^- occurs under ceftriaxone treatment [62]. These cooperative actions are a precondition for the improved synthesis/regeneration of GSH. Similar findings were also present in other experimental conditions [9, 22, 25, 43].

In spite of being significantly beneficial against aluminum neurotoxicity when administered during five consecutive days after the aluminum treatment, these effects of ceftriaxone were moderate in comparison to ceftriaxone pre-treatment. This was most pronounced in the recovery of GSH level, as well as in the activity of cytochrome c oxydase. A slightly better activity of G6PDH than the one achieved in ceftriaxone pre-treatment was not sufficient for GSH recovery. These weaker effects of ceftriaxone in aluminum pre-treatment than in after-treatment are consistent with the already known facts about time-dependent ceftriaxone ability to induce the expression of GLT-1 proteins, system x_c^- and to develop other actions [1, 19, 62]. These results reliably show that ceftriaxone may have therapeutic capabilities, other than preventive, as it has been shown in numerous studies, including our own study stated here.

CONCLUSION

The decreased G6PDH and cytochrome c activity in all the examined brain regions after aluminum application in the CA1 sector of hippocampus, together with the reduced GSH level, suggest an impaired pentose-phosphate metabolism, electron respiratory chain and the synthesis/regeneration of GSH, respectively. These events inevitably lead to the insufficient production of ATP and reducing equivalents whose consequences are the redox disbalance and oxidative stress.

According to the findings related to aluminum neurotoxicity and the protective effects of ceftriaxone against these toxicities, as well as the findings about the predominant role of extracellularly glutamate excess in different models of human diseases, ceftriaxone is one potential therapeutic strategy that could be directed to glutamate clearance. In that aim, the development of drugs that could increase the glutamate clearance by affecting the expression of GLT-1 and system x_c^-, which limits glutamate excitatory actions, could be beneficial. Selectivity must be taken into account due to the EAAT isoforms, as well as their cellular location and relative abundance. Beta-lactam antibiotics, especially the most explored one - ceftriaxone, are a very promising group of drugs in neuroprotection. Their neuroprotective effects, demonstrated both *in vitro* and *in vivo* models, are partly based on the ceftriaxone ability to increase the glutamate uptake and its exchange with cystine, which consequently prevents glutamate excitotoxicity. These pathways should be targets for discovering drugs that could be used in the prevention/treatment of neurodegenerative diseases.

ACKNOWLEDGMENTS

This research was supported by the Ministry of Science of the Republic of Serbia (contract number 143057) and the Ministry of Defense of the Republic of Serbia (contract number MMA/06-10/B.3).

REFERENCES

[1] Rothstein, J.D., Patel, S., Regan, M.R., Haenggeli, C., Huang, Y.H., Bergles, D.E. et al. Beta-lactam antibiotics offer neuroprotection by increasing glutamate transporter expression. *Nature*. 2005; 433(7021):73-7.

[2] Rothstein, J.D., Jin, L., Dykes-Hoberg, M., Kuncl, R.W. Chronic inhibition of glutamate uptake produces a model of slow neurotoxicity. *Proc Natl Acad Sci USA*. 1993; 90(14):6591-5.

[3] Exley, C. Aluminium should now be considered a primary aetiological factor in Alzheimer's disease. *J Alzh Dis Rep*. 2017; 1(1):23-5.

[4] Kawahara, M., Kato-Negishi, M. Link between aluminum and the pathogenesis of Alzheimer's disease: the integration of the aluminum and amyloid cascade hypotheses. *Int J Alzheimers Dis*. 2011; Mar 8; 276393.

[5] Nayak, P., Chatterjee, A.K. Effects of aluminium exposure on brain glutamate and GABA systems: an experimental study in rats. *Food Chem Toxicol*. 2001; 39(12):1285-9.

[6] Redgrove, J., Rodriguez, I., Mahadevan-Bava, S., Exley, C. Prescription infant formulas are contaminated with aluminium. *Int J Environ Res Public Health*. 2019 Mar 12; 16(5). pii: E899. doi: 10.3390/ijerph16050899.

[7] Exley, C. What is the risk of aluminium as a neurotoxin? *Expert Rev Neurother*. 2014; 14(6):589-91.

[8] Zhou, Y., Danbolt, N.C. GABA and glutamate transporters in brain. *Front Endocrinol (Lausanne).* 2013 Nov 11; 4:165. doi: 10.3389/fendo.2013.00165. eCollection 2013.

[9] Rothstein, J.D., Martin, L., Levey, A.I., Dykes-Hoberg, M., Jin, L., Wu, D., Nash, N., Kuncl, R.W. Localization of neuronal and glial glutamate transporters. *Neuron.* 1994; 13:713-25.

[10] Krzyżanowska, W., Pomierny, B., Filip, M., Pera, J. Glutamate transporters in brain ischemia: to modulate or not? *Acta Pharmacol Sin.* 2014; 35(4):444-62.

[11] Rothstein, J.D., Dykes-Hoberg, M., Pardo, C.A., Bristol, L.A., Jin, L., Kuncl, R.W. et al. Knockout of glutamate transporters reveals a major role for astroglial transport in excitotoxicity and clearance of glutamate. *Neuron.* 1996; 16(3):675-86.

[12] Fontana, A.C. Current approaches to enhance glutamate transporter function and expression. *J Neurochem.* 2015; 134(6):982-1007.

[13] Vandenberg, R.J., Ryan, R.M. Mechanisms of glutamate transport. *Physiol Rev.* 2013; 93(4):1621-57.

[14] Ottestad-Hansen, S., Hu, Q.X., Follin-Arbelet, V.V. et al. The cystine-glutamate exchanger (xCT, Slc7a11) is expressed in significant concentrations in a subpopulation of astrocytes in the mouse brain. *Glia.* 2018; 66(5):951-70.

[15] Li, Y., Park, J.S., Deng, J.H., Bai, Y. Cytochrome c oxidase subunit IV is essential for assembly and respiratory function of the enzyme complex. *J Bioenerg Biomembr.* 2006; 38(5-6):283-91.

[16] Wojcik, S.M., Rhee, J.S., Herzog, E., Sigler, A., Jahn, R., Takamori, S. et al. An essential role for vesicular glutamate transporter 1 (VGLUT1) in postnatal development and control of quantal size. *Proc Natl Acad Sci U S A.* 2004; 101(18):7158-63.

[17] Rothstein, J.D., Van Kammen, M., Levey, A.I., Martin, L.J., Kuncl, R.W. Selective loss of glial glutamate transporter GLT-1 in amyotrophic lateral sclerosis. *Ann Neurol.* 1995; 38(1):73-84.

[18] Takahashi, K., Foster, J.B., Lin, C.L. Glutamate transporter EAAT2: regulation, function, and potential as a therapeutic target for

neurological and psychiatric disease. *Cell Mol Life Sci.* 2015; 72(18):3489-506.

[19] Lee, S.G., Su, Z.Z., Emdad, L., Gupta, P., Sarkar, D., Borjabad, A. et al. Mechanism of ceftriaxone induction of excitatory amino acid transporter-2 expression and glutamate uptake in primary human astrocytes. *J Biol Chem.* 2008; 283(19):13116-23.

[20] Ochoa-Aguilar, A., Ventura-Martinez, R., Sotomayor-Sobrino, M.A., Gómez, C., Morales-Espinoza, M.R. Review of antibiotic and non-antibiotic properties of beta-lactam molecules. *Antiinflamm Antiallergy Agents Med Chem.* 2016; 15(1):3-14.

[21] Yimer, E.M., Hishe, H.Z., Tuem, K.B. Repurposing of the β-Lactam Antibiotic, Ceftriaxone for Neurological Disorders: A Review. *Front Neurosci.* 2019 Mar 26; 13:236. eCollection 2019.

[22] Dwivedi, V.K., Bhatanagar, A., Chaudhary, M. Protective role of ceftriaxone plus sulbactam with VRP1034 on oxidative stress, hematological and enzymatic parameters in cadmium toxicity induced rat model. *Interdiscip Toxicol.* 2012; 5(4):192-200.

[23] Altaş, M., Meydan, S., Aras, M., Yılmaz, N., Ulutaş, K.T., Okuyan, H.M., Nacar, A. Effects of ceftriaxone on ischemia/reperfusion injury in rat brain. *J Clin Neurosci.* 2013; 20(3):457-61.

[24] Wei, J., Pan, X., Pei, Z., Wang, W., Qiu, W., Shi, Z., Xiao, G. The beta-lactam antibiotic, ceftriaxone, provides neuroprotective potential via anti-excitotoxicity and anti-inflammation response in a rat model of traumatic brain injury. *J Trauma Acute Care Surg.* 2012; 73(3):654-60.

[25] Lewerenz, J., Albrecht, P., Tien, M.L., Henke, N., Karumbayaram, S., Kornblum, H.I. et al. Induction of Nrf2 and xCT are involved in the action of the neuroprotective antibiotic ceftriaxone in vitro. *J Neurochem.* 2009; 111(2):332-43.

[26] Norris FH. Ceftriaxone in amyotrophic lateral sclerosis. *Arch Neurol.* 1994; 51(5):447.

[27] Ruzza, P., Siligardi, G., Hussain, R., Marchiani, A., Islami, M., Bubacco, L. et al. Ceftriaxone blocks the polymerization of α-

synuclein and exerts neuroprotective effects in vitro. *ACS Chem Neurosci.* 2014; 5(1):30-8.

[28] Zumkehr, J., Rodriguez-Ortiz, C.J., Cheng, D., Kieu, Z., Wai, T., Hawkins, C. et al. Ceftriaxone ameliorates tau pathology and cognitive decline via restoration of glial glutamate transporter in a mouse model of Alzheimer's disease. *Neurobiol Aging.* 2015; 36:2260-71.

[29] Cudkowicz, M.E., Titus, S., Kearney, M., Yu, H., Sherman, A., Schoenfeld, D. et al. Ceftriaxone Study Investigators. Safety and efficacy of ceftriaxone for amyotrophic lateral sclerosis: a multi-stage, randomised, double-blind, placebo-controlled trial. *Lancet Neurol.* 2014; 13(11):1083-91.

[30] Jacob, C.P., Koutsilieri, E., Bartl, J., Neuen-Jacob, E., Arzberger, T., Zander, N. et al. Alterations in expression of glutamatergic transporters and receptors in sporadic Alzheimer's disease. *J Alzheimers Dis.* 2007; 11(1):97-116.

[31] Scimemi, A., Meabon, J.S., Woltjer, R.L., Sullivan, J.M., Diamond, J.S., Cook, D.G. Amyloid-β1-42 slows clearance of synaptically released glutamate by mislocalizing astrocytic GLT-1. *J Neurosci.* 2013; 33(12):5312-8.

[32] Tikhonova, M.A., Amstislavskaya, T.G., Belichenko, V.M., Fedoseeva, L.A., Kovalenko, S.P., Pisareva, E.E. et al. Modulation of the expression of genes related to the system of amyloid-beta metabolism in the brain as a novel mechanism of ceftriaxone neuroprotective properties. *BMC Neurosci.* 2018 Apr 19; 19(Suppl 1):13. doi: 10.1186/s12868-018-0412-5.

[33] Akina, S., Thati, M., Puchchakayala, G. Neuroprotective effect of ceftriaxone and selegiline on scopolamine induced cognitive impairment in mice. *Adv Biol Res.* 2013; 7:266-75.

[34] Kumar, V., Gill, K.D. Oxidative stress and mitochondrial dysfunction in aluminium neurotoxicity and its amelioration: a review. *Neurotoxicology.* 2014; 41:154-66.

[35] Gonçalves, P.P., Silva, V.S. Does neurotransmission impairment accompany aluminium neurotoxicity? *J Inorg Biochem.* 2007; 101(9):1291-338.

[36] Kaur, A., Gill, K.D. Disruption of neuronal calcium homeostasis after chronic aluminium toxicity in rats. *Basic Clin Pharmacol Toxicol.* 2005; 96(2):118-22.

[37] Jelenković, A., Jovanović, M.D., Stevanović, I., Petronijević, N., Bokonjić, D., Zivković, J. et al. Influence of the green tea leaf extract on neurotoxicity of aluminium chloride in rats. *Phytother Res.* 2014; 28(1):82-7.

[38] Tanaka K, Watase K, Manabe T, Yamada, K., Watanabe, M., Takahashi, K. et al. Epilepsy and exacerbation of brain injury in mice lacking the glutamate transporter GLT-1. *Science.* 1997; 276(5319):1699-702.

[39] Petr, G.T., Sun, Y., Frederick, N.M., Zhou, Y., Dhamne, S.C., Hameed, M.Q. et al. Conditional deletion of the glutamate transporter GLT-1 reveals that astrocytic GLT-1 protects against fatal epilepsy while neuronal GLT-1 contributes significantly to glutamate uptake into synaptosomes. *J Neurosci.* 2015; 35(13):5187-201.

[40] Sugimoto, J., Tanaka, M., Sugiyama, K., Ito, Y., Aizawa, H., Soma, M. et al. Region-specific deletions of the glutamate transporter GLT-1 differentially affect seizure activity and neurodegeneration in mice. *Glia.* 2018; 66(4):777-88.

[41] Ulu, M.O., Tanriverdi, T., Oz, B., Biceroglu, H., Isler, C., Eraslan, B.S. et al. The expression of astroglial glutamate transporters in patients with focal cortical dysplasia: an immunohistochemical study. *Acta Neurochir (Wien).* 2010; 152(5):845-53.

[42] Crunelli, V., Carmignoto, G., Steinhäuser, C. Novel astrocyte targets: new avenues for the therapeutic treatment of epilepsy. *Neuroscientist.* 2015; 21(1):62-83.

[43] Hussein, A.M., Ghalwash, M., Magdy, K., Abulseoud, O.A. Beta lactams antibiotic ceftriaxone modulates seizures, oxidative stress and connexin 43 expression in hippocampus of pentylenetetrazole kindled rats. *J Epilepsy Res.* 2016; 6(1):8-15.

[44] Zeng, L.H., Bero, A.W., Zhang, B., Holtzman, D.M., Wong, M. Modulation of astrocyte glutamate transporters decreases seizures in a mouse model of Tuberous Sclerosis Complex. *Neurobiol Dis.* 2010; 37(3):764-71.

[45] Jelenkovic, A.V., Jovanovic, M.D., Stanimirovic, D.D., Bokonjic, D,D., Ocic, G.G., Boskovic, B.S. Beneficial effects of ceftriaxone against pentylenetetrazole-evoked convulsions. *Exp Biol Med (Maywood).* 2008; 233(11):1389-94.

[46] Uyanikgil, Y., Özkeşkek, K., Çavuşoğlu, T., Solmaz, V., Tümer, M.K., Erbas, O. Positive effects of ceftriaxone on pentylenetetrazol-induced convulsion model in rats. *Int J Neurosci.* 2016; 126(1):70-5.

[47] Konig, J.F.R., Klippel, R.A. *The rat brain. A stereotaxic atlas of the forebrain and lower parts of the brain stem.* Baltimore: The Williams and Wilkins Company; 1963.

[48] Bergmeyer, H. *Methods of enzymatic analysis.* New York: Academic Press; 1974.

[49] Hess, H.H., Pope, A. Intralaminar distribution of cytochrome oxidase activity in human frontal isocortex. *J Neurochem.* 1960; 5:207-17.

[50] Anderson, M.E. Tissue glutathione. In: Greenwald, R.A. (ed.). *CRC handbook of methods for oxygen radical research.* Boca Raton: CRC Press; 1985. pp. 317-323.

[51] Saba, K., Rajnala, N., Veeraiah, P., Tiwari, V., Rana, R.K., Lakhotia, S.C., Patel, A.B. Energetics of excitatory and inhibitory neurotransmission in aluminum chloride model of Alzheimer's disease: reversal of behavioral and metabolic deficits by Rasa Sindoor. *Front Mol Neurosci.* 2017 Oct 17; 10:323. doi: 10.3389/fnmol.2017.00323. eCollection 2017.

[52] Walls, A.B., Waagepetersen, H.S., Bak, L.K., Schousboe, A., Sonnewald, U. The glutamine-glutamate/GABA cycle: function, regional differences in glutamate and GABA production and effects of interference with GABA metabolism. *Neurochem Res.* 2015; 40(2):402-9.

[53] Pinky, N.F., Wilkie, C.M., Barnes, J.R., Parsons, M.P. Region- and activity-dependent regulation of extracellular glutamate. *J Neurosci.* 2018; 38(23):5351-66.

[54] Stevanović, I.D., Jovanović, M.D., Colić, M., Ninković, M., Jelenković, A., Mihajlović, R. Cytochrome c oxidase activity and nitric oxide synthase in the rat brain following aluminium intracerebral application. *Folia Neuropathol.* 2013; 51(2):140-6.

[55] Jovanović, M.D., Jelenković, A., Stevanović, I.D., Bokonjić, D., Colić, M., Petronijević, N. et al. Protective effects of glucose-6-phosphate dehydrogenase on neurotoxicity of aluminium applied into the CA1 sector of rat hippocampus. *Indian J Med Res.* 2014; 139:864-72.

[56] Sarti, P., Forte, E., Giuffrè, A., Mastronicola, D., Magnifico, M.C., Arese, M. The chemical interplay between oxide and mitochondrial cytochrome c oxidase: reactions, effectors and pathophysiology. *Int J Cell Biol.* 2012; 2012:571067. doi: 10.1155/2012/571067.

[57] Suárez-Fernández, M.B., Soldado, A.B., Sanz-Medel, A., Vega, J.A., Novelli, A., Fernández-Sánchez, M.T. Aluminum-induced degeneration of astrocytes occurs via apoptosis and results in neuronal death. *Brain Res.* 1999; 835(2):125-36.

[58] Aremu, D.A., Meshitsuka, S. Some aspects of astroglial functions and aluminum implications for neurodegeneration. *Brain Res Rev.* 2006; 52(1):193-200.

[59] Lemire, J., Appanna, V.D. Aluminum toxicity and astrocyte dysfunction: a metabolic link to neurological disorders. *J Inorg Biochem.* 2011; 105(11):1513-7.

[60] Verkhratsky, A., Zorec, R., Rodriguez, J.J., Parpura, V. Pathobiology of neurodegeneration: the role for astroglia. *Opera Med Physiol.* 2016 Jan; 1:13-22.

[61] Stevanović, I.D., Jovanović, M.D., Colić, M., Jelenković, A., Bokonjić, D., Ninković, M. et al. N-nitro-L-arginine methyl ester influence on aluminium toxicity in the brain. *Folia Neuropathol.* 2011; 49:219-29.

[62] Reissner, K.J. The cystine/glutamate antiporter: when too much of a good thing goes bad. *J Clin Invest.* 2014; 124(8):3279-81.

In: Neurological Diseases
Editor: Philip L. Thygesen

ISBN: 978-1-53616-205-9
© 2019 Nova Science Publishers, Inc.

Chapter 3

IMPLEMENTATION OF A CONCEPT OF NEUROPALLIATIVE AND REHABILITATION CARE FOR PATIENTS WITH PROGRESSIVE, NEUROLOGICAL DISEASE IN THE CZECH REPUBLIC: A QUALITATIVE STUDY

Radka Bužgová[1,*], *PhD, Radka Kozáková*[1], *PhD and Michal Bar*[2], *MD, PhD*

[1]Department of Nursing and Midwifery, University of Ostrava, Ostrava, Czech Republic
[2]Neurology Clinic, The University Hospital, Ostrava, Czech Republic

ABSTRACT

Palliative care provided to patients with progressive neurological disease (PND) can result in an improvement of the quality of their life. The aim of the qualitative research was to propose an implementation of a

---

[*] Corresponding Author's Email: radka.buzgova@osu.cz.

concept of neuropalliative and rehabilitation care for patients with PND within the system of health- and social care in the Czech Republic. The research included focus groups (n = 4) comprising 33 participants. The method of thematic analysis was used to analyze the obtained data. The research included 33 participants - 30 professionals working with PND patients, 2 hospital chaplains, and a patient with PD. A three-level model was suggested consisting of the following phases: 1/ supportive care / rehabilitation, 2/ neuropalliative rehabilitation, 3/ specialist palliative care. Efficient communication methods, support of the family, and identification of suitable patients were emphasized in the individual phases of provided care. For further research, we recommend verifying the efficiency of the three-level concept of the neuropalliative and rehabilitation care in an intervention study.

Keywords: dying, quality of life, neurology, rehabilitation, support, palliative care

INTRODUCTION

In 2008, the European Association for Palliative Care launched a discussion about the development of palliative care for patients with neurological diseases. Together with the European Academy of Neurology (EAN) they have engaged in improving the cooperation of the palliative and neurological care providers. Their aim is to improve the care secured to people with progressive neurological diseases – PND (Borasio, Sloan and Pongratz 1998). The concept of neuropalliative and rehabilitation care suitable for e.g., patients with multiple sclerosis (MS), Parkinson's disease (PD), motor neuron disease (MND), or Huntington's disease is defined by Sutton (2008) as "a holistic approach to the care of neurological patients with significant disability, complex needs, and a potentially shortened life-span. It is patient-centered and involves diagnosis of clinical problems at all stages, rehabilitation to maintain function, care coordination and appropriate palliation to relieve symptoms." (National Council for Palliative Care 2007). Oliver et al. (2016) based review recommended the early integration of palliative care, multidisciplinary team care, communication, symptom management, carer support, ends-of-life care, including the wish for hastened death for people with progressive neurological diseases.

According to the palliative care standards (Sláma, Kabelka and Špinková 2013), in the Czech Republic the patients with PND represent one of the target groups of the palliative care. However, there is no concept designed to interconnect the palliative and neurological care. According to the available statistics of the National Database of Palliative Care (Švancara, Sláma and Kabelka 2016) between 2011 and 2015 most Czech patients with PND died in a hospital, especially patients with the motor neuron disease (54%), and sclerosis multiplex (54%). Only a few of these patients died in a hospice – most of them were people with motor neuron disease (8%). A greater amount of hospitalizations during the final year of life was registered among patients who died in a health-care facility. Recently, the authors pointed out the lack of knowledge about the efficiency and usability of the palliative care for patients with PND, e.g., patients with PD (Richfield, Jones and Alty 2013; Lennaerts, Groot and Steppe 2017) even though research shows that the palliative care alleviate the symptoms and improves the quality of life of people with PND. After introducing palliative care, patients with ALS, MS, and PD reported improved life quality as well as less pain, dyspnea, sleep disorders, and intestinal symptoms (Veronese et al. 2015). Palliative care in the Czech Republic included in the health-care system is currently available mainly to the patients with oncological diseases. The Czech health-care system is based on obligatory public insurance. The residence and mobile hospice care is paid through the public health insurance; however, the patients with PND usually fail to pass the conditions to be repaid (difficult estimate of the disease progress), (Bužgová, Kozáková and Juríčková 2019a).

Under the project of the Czech Health Research Council of the Czech Ministry of Health (AZV MZ CR), we studied the most common unfulfilled needs of patients with PND and their relatives with the aim to design a concept of care for these patients. Among the most frequent unfulfilled needs of the patients were problems with the adaptation to the disease (difficulties when arranging basic matters, social isolation, acceptance of the limitations resulting from the disease, coping with the negative emotions, problems with utilizing one's leisure time), as well as those caused by insufficient professional help (lack of information, control of symptoms, obstacles when outside one's home, insufficient equipment, problems when securing the care including rehabilitation, maintaining human dignity, and use of optimum interventions at the end of life), (Bužgová, Kozáková and Sikorová 2018; Bužgová, Kozáková and Juríčková 2019a).

Regarding the relatives, the most frequent unmet needs that were identified included the lack of information, high demands on the caring family, insufficient support of the health- and social workers, problems when securing health- and social care, and problems when securing the care at the end of life (Bužgová, Kozáková and Juríčková 2019b).

Based on the identified unmet needs of patients and their relatives and through an analysis of expert discussions the aim of this research was to suggest an implementation of a concept of neuropalliative and rehabilitation care for patients with progressive neurological disease into the system of health- and social care in the Czech Republic.

METHODS

The authors opted for the methodology of qualitative research using the thematic analysis method (Braun and Clarke 2006). Palliative care is a field ripe for the application of qualitative research (Lim et al. 2017). The study met COREQ criteria for reporting of qualitative research (Tong, Sainsbury and Craig 2007).

Participants

The research included 33 participants - 30 professionals working with PND patients, 2 hospital chaplains, and a patient with PD (see Table 1). The selection of the participants was intentional according to the given criteria: 1. professionals – professional qualification to perform the specified profession, experience with care for patients with progressive neurological disease lasting at least 1 year, signed informed consent; 2. patients: diagnosis of the progressive neurological disease (PD, MS, MND or HD), at least 1 year after the diagnosis was stated, age > 18 years, Mini Mental State Exam (MMSE) ≥ 24 ponts, signed informed consent.

Tale 1. Characteristics of participants

Participants:	N	age	practice	gender
Patients with Parkinson's disease	1	72	---	M
Medical doctor – neurologist	3	41-64	14-38	F, 2M
Medical doctor – palliative medicine	1	57	32	F
Medical doctor – rehabilitation	1	54	28	F
Nurse – long term care	4	29-58	9-35	4 F
Nurse – hospital	4	29-64	7-42	4 F
Nurse – community care, ambulance	7	27-42	5-19	7 F
Physiotherapist	3	26-45	4-25	3 F
Ergotherapist	2	29-39	6-15	2 F
Social worker	3	41-42	18-21	3 F
Psychologist	2	35-40	4-15	2 F
Hospital chaplain	2	45-68	15-24	2 M

We selected healthcare professionals with professional competence and experience of care of patients with PND in hospital, health or social facilities, or home care. Ideally, participants should reflect a range of ages, levels, professions (medical doctor, nurse, social worker, physiotherapist, ergotheapist, psychologist, hospital chaplain) and patterns of working. The method of obtaining the sample was the snow ball technique. The remainder of the participants were selected according to recommendations from the studies individuals. Emphasis was placed on participants' experience of the specified topic. Participants were accepted until theoretical saturation of the sample was achieved (theoretical sampling = data collection based on emerging hypotheses from the ongoing analysis). Potential participants were contacted directly by RB (health professionals) and RK (patient) by email or phone. To meet the needs of theoretical sampling, and achieve theoretical saturation, diversity was sought in experience of PND disease (patient), and in experience of care of patients with PND (healthcare professionals): i.e., disease type, age, location, and number of years making diagnoses or caring for people with PND. Diversity was also sought in type of facilities (hospitals, nursing homes, social facilities, rehabilitation facilities, home care) and their size and location.

Data Collection

The chosen method of data collection were focus groups (n = 4). Each of the focus groups included 8-9 participants. Written informed consent was obtained at the start of each group, following further explanation of the study by the researchers, and an opportunity for participants to ask questions. The focus groups were facilitated by a researcher (RB). The focus groups discussed the experiences of experts with the given topic. The participants were asked two basic questions:

- What are your ideas about the possibility of applying palliative care to patients in advanced stage of neurological disease and in what phase should it be introduced?
- Which way would it be possible to apply the concept of neuropalliative and rehabilitation care in the Czech Republic?

Each focus group lasted for 120 minutes. All focus groups were recorded on a voice recorder, and subsequently transcribed verbatim. The focus group setting can help the participants share their perspectives on novel care paradigm (Lim et al. 2017) which the concept of neuropalliative and rehabilitation care is. The focus group guide questions were thoroughly discussed and refined by the research group in advance. The focus group guide was adapted accordingly for the subsequent follow-up discussions based on the previous responses and ongoing data analysis. All four group sessions took place at the University of Ostrava, Faculty of Medicine.

The data were collected under the qualitative research of the Czech Ministry of Health research project no. 17-29447A titled "Neuropalliative and rehabilitation approach to maintain the quality of life of patients in an advanced stage of specific neurological diseases." The study conforms to the provisions of the Declaration of Helsinki and was approved by the ethics committee of University Hospital Ostrava (no. 486/2016).

Data Analysis

The focus groups were recorded on a voice recorder and, afterwards, literally transcribed. The acquired data were then organized and described in detail through thematic analysis. The thematic analysis is based on moving back and forth among the individual data segments, among the extracts, and data codes, and their analysis. The analysis was performed in five phases (Hendl, 2016):

1. Acquainting with the data. Two researchers (RB, RK) independently codified the raw transcript.
2. Generating initial codes.
3. Theme search. Analysis of codes and data to suggest wider meaning patterns (potential themes).
4. Elaborating the topics and their revision.
5. Defining and naming the themes.
6. Preparation of the report. Connecting the analytical narration and data extracts and contextualization with the current literature.

RESULTS

The elements of palliative care can be used early on when determining the diagnosis, particularly with respect to the manner of the doctor's communication with the patient or the family about the disease and its progress. Both the patient and his/her family should be provided appropriate support when adapting to the diagnosed disease. At the same time, the neurological treatment is secured including the diagnostics, examination, and therapy leading to the alleviation of the symptoms.

The suggested model of neuropalliative and rehabilitation care may be applied to patients with aggravating symptoms where their self-sufficiency is gradually limited (Palliative Performance Scale PPS < 70). Since the various neurological diseases progress with different speed, the period after stating the diagnosis may vary.

Based on the discussion of the focus groups, a three-level model was designed including the palliative and neurological care in the following stages: 1/ supportive care and complex rehabilitation, 2/ neuropalliative rehabilitation, 3/ specialized palliative care. All levels include multidisciplinary professional care completed with informal help and the help of patient organizations to support the care for the patient in his or her home environment (see Figure 1).

MULTIDISCIPLINARY PROFESSIONAL CARE
informal helps / patients organizations / domestic support

SYMPTOM MANAGEMENT -	neurology care	neurology/palliative	special palliative team
PERSONAL CARE/HYGIENE -	support for self-sufficiency	care/accepting dependence	dignity
ACTIVITY OF DAILY LIVING -	low support	medium support	high support
PSYCHOSOCIAL-WELLBEING –	support with acceptance of illness	coping with emotions	good death
SOCIAL SUPPORT –	health-social services and financial benefits counseling	aids	place of care
MOBILITY/TRANSPORT -	by himself/low support	support	support
RELATIONSHIPS –	support with family relationships	family communication about end-of-life care plan	
COMMUNICATION –	diagnosis • progression • health/social care • living wills • end-of life care • grief		
REHABILITATION -	active	active/passive	passive
CAREGIVER SUPPORT -	low	medium/respite care	high

CO-ORDINATOR OF CARE

Social rehabilitation and physiotherapy → Neuropalliative rehabilitation → Specialist palliative care

Neurology treatment

Supportive care

DIAGNOSIS — **DEATH** — **BEREVEMENT**

Figure 1. Model of care for patients with progressive neurological disease.

1. Supportive Care and Complex Rehabilitation

The aim of the supportive care is improved self-sufficiency and quality of life of the patient with maximized abilities and involvement of the patient in the treatment and care. The neurological treatment should focus on the reduction of symptoms (pain and other symptoms leading to suffering) and helping with the patient's discomfort.

Rehabilitation includes the treatment of physical problems (physiotherapy, ergo therapy), psychological difficulties (psychotherapy, cognitive rehabilitation), and social support (consulting social benefits and services). The patient should be properly informed about the disease; all options of treatment in the individual phases of the disease should be explained to the patient. The doctor should get the information over to the patient gradually, step by step, right from the onset of the disease. It is important to gradually inform the family members about the possibilities of care so that in case of need they know where to go for help. The aim of providing the information is also to support the patient and the relatives so that they are aware that they will be looked after during all stages of the disease.

As a part of the supportive care, a care coordinator should be determined, who would cooperate with the doctor – neurologist and the general practitioner who cares for patients with PND. It would be convenient to compile a register of patients which the coordinator would be able to access. All care for the patient should start at home; after that, the options of institutional care should be considered.

Within the rehabilitation care, functional goals should be determined, e.g., whether the patients will be able to look after themselves in the bed, will be able to cross the room, will be able to go to the restroom on their own, maintain personal hygiene on their own. Furthermore, all barriers of self-sufficiency should be identified, all limits, all areas that may improve. Physiotherapy could be secured in the rehabilitation institute or spa service. It is necessary that it continues within the outpatient care. The doctors themselves stated that the neurological examination describes e.g., serious paresis, hemiparesis, but not the prospects of the individual (e.g., whether the person will learn to walk). There the cooperation of the neurologist and the rehabilitation doctor is very beneficial.

It is also appropriate to secure some psychological help. The patients expect some communication with the psychologist and his or her help with processing their emotions, or possibly educating the family members.

In case of complicated symptoms, there may be required a consultation with a palliative doctor to alleviate the symptoms of the disease. The patient and his or her family should be offered the possibility to consult the care plan at the end of life, goals of treatment, or to write down previously mentioned wishes in the early stage of the disease.

2. Neuropalliative Rehabilitation

It is intended for patients in advanced stage of disease when any improvement is not possible (PPS ≤ 50). The goal is to maintain the physical condition and cognitive abilities, or possibly to slow down the loss of self-sufficiency. In this phase, it is possible to review the plan of the end of life and the previously expressed wishes or to write them down in case the patient or the family members did not discuss this topic earlier. The multidisciplinary team should support the family with respect to mutual communication about the progressing disease.

At this stage, a regular evaluation should be performed by the multidisciplinary team within the outpatient care (doctor, nurse, speech therapist, physiotherapist, psychiatrist, psychologist, social worker, ergo therapist). It is good to start with breathing rehabilitation very early on, even before any development of breathing difficulties (particularly for patients with ALS). Furthermore, the ergo therapist and physiotherapist should focus on spasticity and locomotion, appropriate equipment should be secured on time, the speech therapist should focus on the possibility of alternative communication in case of speech problems, and the psychological care should support coping with emotions, social changes, and increasing dependence on the help of others, including the support of maintaining human dignity. The patients and the relatives should during the checkups get support from the multidisciplinary team also due to the social isolation. When the patient is not able to come to the health facility because of the advancing disease, the care should be provided at his or her home. The participants of our research agreed that currently the patients are cared for in their home environment only rarely. The care coordinator cooperating with the general practitioner should play a crucial role. Any care at home of the client should be provided by a home care agency, care service, or mobile hospice. In case of substantial deterioration of the cognitive functions, it is necessary to secure the patient's representative and the place where the care is provided in accordance with the patient's wish and the possibilities of the family.

Due to the progress of the disease and increased dependence of the patient on the care of other people, it is appropriate to secure some alleviation services – both at home of the patient and in the form of a contemporary stay of the patient in a different facility. Courses for the caring relatives ideally in their homes are also helpful. If it is not possible to provide the care at home of the patient it is necessary to secure appropriate institutional care in a social services facility (for people under 60 years of age – specialized homes for people with progressive neurological disease, for people over 60 years of age – homes for seniors, homes with special regime).

3. Specialized Palliative Care

Specialized palliative care is intended for patients in advanced and terminal stage of the disease with the aim of providing comfort, to maximize the quality of life, and minimize the burden of the illness on the patient as well as his or her family. The goal is not to restore one's health or improve the state, but to improve the quality of the final part of the patient's life and to provide the so called "nice death". According to the patients themselves, nice death mainly means the death without pain, securing one's privacy, and social contact with the others.

What is a problem is especially determining the final phase of the disease for the patients with PND. The focus group participants agreed on the following criteria for determining the time for transition to the specialized palliative care for patients with PND:

- No treatment works,
- The disease is progressing substantially although the death prognosis is not clear,
- Deterioration of the physical symptoms of the disease,
- Distinct setback of the functional state,
- Breathing and swallowing difficulties,
- Decrease of self-sufficiency leading to full dependency on the care.

Another important aspect should be the wish of the patient or the family to secure the services of the specialized palliative care.

The patients in the final stage of life also need the multidisciplinary care. Besides the above-mentioned members of the multidisciplinary team, there should also be an expert from the sleep center, or lung doctor (particularly for patients with ALS with artificial ventilation). The rehabilitation should continue, possibly only the passive rehabilitation to maintain the self-sufficiency.

The care should be primarily provided in the home environment of the client, if it is possible. The patient should have proper aids and equipment available (e.g., adjustable bed) and should be supported by the multidisciplinary team (including a physiotherapist), mobile hospice care.

In case of excessive burden to the family or impossibility of home care for other reasons, institutional care should be secured in a social services facility or in a hospice. If the patient stayed in a social services facility before, he or she should be provided the care in the same facility or through the services of the mobile hospice care.

The family should be provided support and consultancy about the place of care at the end of life and the support to accept such decision. The hospice care is suitable for patients with respiration insufficiency or patients who need palliative sedation, who cannot have for some reason the non-invasive ventilation, or substantially suffer from breathlessness (particularly patients with ALS).

Part of the specialized palliative care is also the support of the family after the patient's death.

DISCUSSION

Procuring the so called early palliative care is the new paradigm of the palliative care (Lim et al. 2017). The reason is the existing evidence that confirm the improved results of care for patients with oncological disease (Temel et al. 2010; Zimmermann et al. 2014; Temel et al. 2017). Timely introduction of palliative care is therefore recommended for patients with PND as well (Oliver, Borasio, and Caraceni 2016; Dallara and Tolchin 2014) where the symptom management improves together with the satisfaction of patients and their families (Edmonds et al. 2010; Higginson et al. 2009). Waldron et al. (2013) pointed out that professionals often overlook the relevance of the palliative care.

The time of launching the palliative care differs according to the basic diagnosis and the progress of the disease. For instance, the average length of life with ALS is 3 to 5 years. The symptoms and handicaps that the patients suffer may be quite serious and may develop early on after determining the diagnosis. Therefore, palliative care should be launched for this disease right after the diagnosis is ascertained. Patients with PD, on the other hand, live on average for 15 years and palliative care should be introduced sometime during the development of the disease (Veronese and Oliver 2013).

The chronic, continually deteriorating motoric handicap however results for all patients with PND in a range of health as well as psychosocial problems both for the patient and his or her family and it requires multidisciplinary care and cooperation (Bužgová, Kozáková and Juríčková 2019a; Bužgová, Kozáková and Juríčková 2019b). Based on the findings of our research, we recommend applying a three-level model interlinking the supportive, palliative, and neurological care. A multidisciplinary team where all members contribute to the close cooperation with others with their expertise should secure and provide the assessment and care for patients. The team should represent at least the following professions: doctor, nurse, social worker, and psychologist/ counsellor. The team may be expanded to include other experts like physiotherapists, ergo therapists, nutritional therapists, and speech therapists (Oliver et al. 2016). Available studies declare the efficiency of the multidisciplinary approach, particularly in case of care for people with ALS (Aridegbe et al. 2013; Rooney et al. 2015) and MS (Edmonds et al. 2010). The care for patients with PND is usually long-term and needs to be coordinated by a single person. One of the solutions may be the graduates of a new graduate study program in the Czech Republic titled Coordination of rehabilitation and long-term care. This field of study should prepare the experts with multidisciplinary knowledge and skills who would be able to identify, suggest, negotiate, and perform sets of multidisciplinary measures to solve the consequences of altered physical condition of people suffering from long-term disease.

An important recommendation of our research is the use of communication techniques common for the palliative care (e.g., how to convey the diagnosis and negative news to the patient) for all patients right after determining the diagnosis. The research suggests that the doctor's communication is often insufficient or inefficient especially with respect to newly diagnosed patients (O'Brien et al. 2011; Aoun et al. 2012).

It is well known that communication with patients and their families is very important within the palliative care and there are studies that demonstrate that clear and open communication improves the care for people with PND (Borasio 2013). There might appear specific problems when communicating with people with PND which result from the pathological processes that progress with varying speed and which usually combine the cognitive function disorder and speech difficulties. Timely planning of future care is particularly recommended for these types of disease when the progress of the disease may lead to deteriorated communication and cognitive abilities. The planning of future care should start when the patient is still able to communicate his or her wishes and preferences and can possibly write down the previously expresses desires (Hussain, Adams and Campbell 2013). This might help when providing care to the person later (Jacobsen et al. 2011). According to Buecken, Galushko and Golla (2012), patients with MS expressed their wish to discuss the progress of their illness with their doctors.

Another important recommendation of our research is to include the patient's family in the care as well. Caring for people with PND often results in substantial burden to the caregivers and may bring about a range of negative physical, psychological, social, and financial consequences. Reconciliation with the loss of functional abilities linked to the neurological disease and the impacts of these losses may result in depression and lowered quality of life of the caregivers (Miyashita et al. 2009). The caring family should be supported throughout the whole time when they face the disease. There is evidence that regular evaluation of the caregivers' needs and provided support lower not only the strain of the caregivers but also the negative effects of long-term care (Miyashita et al. 2009; Trail et al. 2003). According to Aarslanda et al. (1999), it is particularly difficult for the caregivers to cope with the changes of cognitive abilities of their relatives which appear in the later stages of many neurological diseases. Psychosocial support and counseling of the caregivers is imperative even after the patient dies (Kissane et al. 2006) and should be aimed at the wider family as well. In the same way, the long-lasting role of a caregiver and his or her confrontation with the increasing physical dependence and cognitive changes of patients (Pereira, Fonseca and Carvalho 2011) require supportive care. Appropriate advice, education, and support may lower the risk of burn-out and emotional suffering (Melo and Oliver 2011; Fillion et al. 2009).

Another significant topic is the study of suitable criteria for the identification of patients where the specialized palliative care should be started. Identifying the progress of the disease leading to the end of the patient's life is crucial so that the patients and their families can be provided appropriate care and support (Neudert, Wasner and Borasio 2001). The following indicators were suggested to recognize the coming end of life of patients with PND: no treatment works, the disease is substantially progressing, although the prognosis of death is not clear, deterioration of physical symptoms, distinct decline of functional state, breathing and swallowing difficulties, lower self-sufficiency leading to full dependence on the caregiver. According to the criteria of end of life care in long term

(National End of Life Care Programme 2010) there were also included the recurrent infections, cognitive disorders, and loss of weight. According to Hussaina et al. (2014), these indicators may contribute to determine the end of life. Richfield et al. (2013) state that regarding the patients with PD, the specialized palliative care should be considered in case of weight loss, and decreased effectivity of the treatment. The symptoms and other problems may be efficiently solved by the multidisciplinary team experienced in expert palliative care (Bausewein et al. 2014). Patients with PND in the terminal stage of disease should be provided some of the forms of specialized palliative care.

CONCLUSION

In conclusion, to improve the care for patients with PND, we recommend the application of a three-level model of neuropalliative and rehabilitation care. The duration of providing care in the individual phases may vary according to the type of the disease and its progress. What needs to be emphasized is the efficient communication, support of family members, and provision of specialized palliative care in the terminal stage of the illness. For further research, we recommend verifying the efficiency of the three-level concept of the neuropalliative and rehabilitation care in an intervention study.

ACKNOWLEDGMENTS

The study was funded by the Ministry of Health, Czech Republic (no. AZV MZ ČR no. 17-29447A - "A neuropalliative rehabilitation approach to preserve the quality of life in patients with an advanced stage of selected neurological diseases").

REFERENCES

Aarsland, D., Larsen, J.P., Karlsen, K., Lim, N.G., and Tandberg, E. 1999. Mental symptoms in Parkinson's disease are important contributors to caregiver distress. *International Journal of Geriatric Psychiatry* 14:866-874.

Aoun, S.M., Connors, S.L., Priddis, L., Breen, L.J., and Colyer, S. 2012. Motor Neurone Disease family carers' experiences of caring, palliative care and bereavement: An exploratory qualitative study. *Palliative Medicine* 26:842-850.

Aridegbe, T., Kandler, R., Walters, S.J., Walsh, T., Shaw, P.J., and McDermott, C.J. 2013. The natural history of motor neuron disease: Assessing the impact of specialist care. *Amyotrophics Lateral Sclerosis & Frontotemporal Degeneration* 14(1):13-19. doi: 10.3109/17482968.2012.690419.

Bausewein, C., Hau, P., Borasio, G.D., and Voltz, R. 2003. How do patients with primary brain tumours die? *Palliative Medicine* 17(6):558-559. doi: 10.1177/026921630301700615.

Borasio, G.D., Sloan, R., and Pongratz, D.E. 1998. Breaking the news in amyotrophic lateral sclerosis. *Journal of Neurology Science* 160(suppl 1): S127–S133.

Borasio, G.D. 2013. The role of palliative care in patients with neurological disease. Nature Reviews. *Neurology* 9(5):292–295. doi: 10.1038/nrneurol.2013.49.

Braun, V., and Clarke, V. 2006. Using thematic analysis in psychology. *Qualitative Research in Psychology* 3(2):77-101. doi: 10.1191/1478088706qp063oa.

Buecken, R., Galushko, M., and Golla, H. 2012. Patients feeling severely affected by multiple sclerosis: How do patients want to communicate about end-of-life issues? *Patient Education and Counseling* 88:318–324.

Bužgová, R., Kozáková, R., and Sikorová, L. 2018. The unmet palliative care needs of patients with an advanced stage of selected neurological diseases in the Czech Republic. *Palliative Medicine* 32:162.

Bužgová, R., Kozáková, R., and Juríčková, L. 2019a. The unmet needs of patients with progressive neurological diseases in the Czech republic: A qualitative study. *Journal of Palliative Care* 34(1):38-46. doi: 10.1177/0825859718800489.

Bužgová, R., Kozáková, R., and Juríčková, L. 2019b. The unmet needs of family members of patients with progressive neurological disease in the Czech Republic. *Plos One* 14:1-17.

Dallara, A., and Tolchin Weiss, D. 2014. Emerging Subspecialties in Neurology: Palliative care. *Neurology* 82:640–642.

Edmonds, P., Hart, S., Wei Gao, Bibat, B., Burman, R., Silber, R., and Higginson, I.J. 2010. Palliative care for people severely affected by multiple sclerosis: Evaluation of a novel palliative care service. *Multiple Sclerosis* 16(1): 627-636. doi: 10.1177/1352458510364632.

Fillion, L., Duval, S., Dumont, S., Gagnon, P., Tremblay, I. Bairati, I., and Breibart, W.S. 2009. Impact of a meaning-centered intervention on job satisfaction and on quality of life among palliative care nurses. *Psychooncology* 18(12):1300-1310. doi: 10.1002/pon.1513.

Hendl, J. 2016. *Qualitative research. Basic theory, methods and applications*. Praha: Portál.

Higginson, I.J., McCrone, P., Hart, S.R., Burman, R., Silber, E., and Edmonds, P.M. 2009. Is short-term palliative care cost effective in multiple sclerosis. A randomized phase II trial. *Journal of Pain and Symptom Manage* 38(6):816-826. doi: 10.1016/j.jpainsymman.2009.07.002.

Hussain, J., Adams, D., and Campbell, C. 2013. End-of-life care in neurodegenerative conditions: Outcomes of a specialist palliative neurology service. *International Journal of Palliative Nursing* 19:162–169. doi.org/10.12968/ijpn.2013.19.4.162.

Hussain, J.A., Adams, D., Allgar, V., and Campbell, C. 2014. Triggers in advanced neurological conditions: Prediction and management of the terminal phase. *BMJ Supportive Palliative Care* 4(1):30-37. doi: 10.1136/bmjspcare-2012-000389.

Jacobsen, J., Robinson, E., Jackson, V.A., Meiqs, J.B., and Billings, J.A. 2011. Development of a Cognitive Model for Advance Care Planning

Discussions: Results from a Quality Improvement Initiative. *Journal of Palliative Medicine* 14(3): 331-336. doi: 10.1089/jpm.2010.0383.

Kissane, D.W., McKenzie, M., Bloch, S., Moskowitz, C., McKenzie, D.P., and O'Neill, I. 2006. Family focused grief therapy: A randomized, controlled trial in palliative care and bereavement. *American Journal of Psychiatry* 163(7):1208–1218.

Lennaerts, H., Groot, M., and Steppe M. 2017. Palliative care for patients with Parkinson's disease: Study protocol for a mixed methods study. *BMC Palliative Care* 16:61. doi: 10.1186/s12904-017-0248-2.

Lim, T., Tadmor, A., Fujisawa, D., MacDonald, J.J., Gallagher, E.R., Eusebio, J., and Park, E.R. 2017. Qualitative research in palliative care: Applications to clinical trials work. *Journal of palliative medicine* 20(8):857-861.

Melo, C.G., and Oliver, D. 2011. Can addressing death anxiety reduce health care workers' burnout and improve patient care? *Journal of Palliative Care* 27(4): 287–295.

Miyashita, M., Narita, Y., Sakamoto, A., Kawada, N., Akiyama, M., Kayama, M., Suzukamo, Y., and Fukuhara, S. 2009. Care burden and depression in caregivers caring for patients with intractable neurological diseases at home in Japan. *Journal of Neurology Science* 276(1-2): 148–152.

National Council for Palliative Care. 2007. *Focus on Neurology: Addressing Palliative Care for People with Neurological Conditions*. NCPC: London.

National End of Life Care Programme. 2010. *End of Life Care in Long Term Neurological Conditions: A Framework for Implementation*.

Neudert, C., Wasner, M., and Borasion, G.D. 2001. Patients' assessment of quality of life instruments: A randomized study of SIP, SF-36 and SEIQoL-DW in patients with amyotrophic lateral sclerosis. *Journal of Neurology Science* 191(1-2): 103-109.

O'Brien, M.R., Whitehead, B., Jack, B.A.. and Mitchell, J.D. 2011. From symptom onset to a diagnosis of amyotrophic lateral sclerosis/motor neuron disease (ALS/MND and family carers – a qualitative study. *Amyotrophic Lateral Sclerosis* 12:97-104.

Oliver, D.J., Borasio, G.D., and Caraceni, A. 2016. A consensus review on the development of palliative care for patients with chronic and progressive neurological disease. *European Journal of Neurology* 23(1):30-38. doi: 10.1111/ene.12889.

Oliver, D.J., Borasio, G.D., Caraceni, A., de Visser M., Grisold, W., Lorenzl, S., Veronese, S, Voltz, R. 2016. Palliative care in chronic and progressive neurological disease: Summary of a consensus review. *European Journal of Palliative Care* 23(5): 232-235.

Pereira, S.M., Fonseca, A.M., and Carvalho, A.S. 2011. Burnout in palliative care: A systematic review. *Nursing Ethics* 18(3):317–326. doi: 10.1177/0969733011398092.

Richfield, E.W., Jones, E.J., and Alty, J. 2013. Palliative care for Parkinson's disease: A summary of the evidence and future directions. *Palliative Medicine* 27(9):805-810. doi: 10.1177/0269216313495287.

Rooney, J., Byrne, S., Heverin, M., Tobin, K., Dick, A., and Donaghy, C. 2015. A multidisciplinary clinic approach improves survival in ALS: A comparative study of ALS in Ireland and Northern Ireland. *Journal of neurology, neurosurgery and psychiatry* 86(5):496-501. doi: 10.1136/jnnp-2014-309601.

Sláma, O., Kabelka, L., and Špinková, M. 2013. *Palliative care in CR in year 2013*. Praha a Brno: Perspektiva České společnosti paliativní medicíny ČLS JEP.

Sutton, L. 2008. Addressing palliative and end-of-life care needs in neurology. *British Journal of Neuroscience Nursing* 4:235-238.

Švancara, J., Sláma, O., and Kabelka, L. 2016. *The National Data Basis for Palliative Care*. Praha: National Health Information System CR.

Temel, J.S., Greer, J.A., Muzikansky, E., Gallagher, E.R., Admane, S., Jackson, V.A., Dahlin, C.M., Blinderman, C.D., Jacobsen, J., Pirl, W.F., Bilings, J.A., and Lynch, T.J. 2010. Early palliative care for patients with metastatic non-small-cell lung cancer. *The New England journal of medicine* 363(8):733-742. doi: 10.1056/NEJMoa1000678.

Temel, J.S., Greer, J.A., El-Jawahri, A., Pirl, E.R., Park, E.R., Jackson, V.A., Back, A.L., Kamdar, M., Jacobsen, J., Chittenden E.H., Rinaldi, S.P., Gallagher, E.R., Eusebio, J.R., Li, Z., Muzikansky, A., and Ryan, D.P.

2017. Effects of early palliative care in patients with lung and gastrointestinal cancer: A randomized clinical Trial. *Journal of Clinical Oncology* 35(8):834-841. doi: 10.1200/JCO.2016.70.5046.

Tong, A., Sainsbury, P., and Craig, J. (2007). Consolidated criteria for reporting qualitative research (COREQ): A 32-item check list for interviews and focus groups. *International Journal of Quality in Health Care*. 19:349-357.

Trail, M., Nelson, N.D., Van, J.N., Appel, S.H., and Lai EC. 2003. A study comparing patients with amyotrophic lateral sclerosis and their caregivers on measures of quality of life, depression, and their attitudes toward treatment options. *Journal of Neurology Science* 209(1-2):79–85.

Veronese, S., and Oliver, D. 2013. *Palliative Care for People with Neurodegenerative Conditions*. LAP Lambert Academic Publishing.

Veronese, S., Gallo, G., Valle, A., Cugno, C., Chio, A., Calvo, A., Cavalla, P., Zibetti, M., Rivoiro, C., and Oliver, D.J. 2015. Specialist palliative care improves the quality of life in advanced neurodegenerative disorders: NE-PAL, a pilot randomised controlled study. *BMJ Supportive Palliative Care* 7(2):164-172. doi: 10.1136/bmjspcare-2014-000788.

Waldron, M., Kernohan, W.H., Hasson, F., Foster, S., and Cochrane, B. 2013. What do social workers think about the palliative care needs of people with Parkinson's disease? *British Journal of Social Work* 43:81-98. doi:10.1093/bjsw/bcr157.

Zimmermann, C., Swami, N., Krzyzanowka, M., Hannon, B., Leighl, N., Oza, A. Moore, M., Rydall, A., Rodin, G., Tannock, I., Donner, A., and Lo, C. 2014. Early palliative care for patients with advance cancer: A cluster randomized controlled trial. *Lancet* 383(9930):1721-1730. doi: 10.1016/S0140-6736(13)62416-2.

BIOGRAPHICAL SKETCH

Radka Bužgová

Affiliation: Department of Nursing and Midwifery, Faculty of Medicine, University of Ostrava

Education: BSc., Health-social and geriatric care, Medical-Social Faculty, Ostrava University (1997); MSc, Social politic and social work, Pedagogical faculty, University Hradec Králové (2001); Ph.D., Specialization in Health Service, Prevention, Rehabilitation and Therapeutic Care for Children, Adults and Seniors. Faculty of Health and Social Studies, University of South Bohemia in České Budějovice (2009); PhDr., Rehabilitation psychosocial care for disabled children, adults and seniors, Faculty of Health and Social Studies, University of South Bohemia in České Budějovice (2013); Doc., Social medicine, Faculty of Medicine, Palacký university, Olomouc (2016).

Business Address: Syllabova 19, Ostrava 700 30, Czech Republic

Research and Professional Experience: Research focus: health related quality of life, psychometric properties of scales, acceptability of treatment, the impact of treatment on the quality of life, self-esteem and depression, needs assessment, death and dying, palliative care. 25 articles in journals with impact factor, 67 articles in journals in SCOPUS, 3 books (2 first author), 12 articles in peer-review journals.

Working practice: Institute of social care for physically handicapped people in Hrabyně, social therapist (1997-1999); Diakonie ČCE Ostrava, Social service centre for children from crisis family and social service center for seniors, the head of the centre 1999-2005); a lecturer at the Department of Nursing and Midwifery, Faculty of Medicine, Ostrava University (2006 – so far); Mobile hospice Ondrášek, Ostrava (2012 – so far).

Professional Appointments: assistant professor

Honors: Dean's Award for best published work in non-medical fields per year 2011 "Violation of ethical principles in institutional care for older people."

Publications from the Last 3 Years:

Bužgová R., Kozáková, R., Sikorová, L., et al. Measuring quality of life of cognitively impaired elderly inpatients in palliative care: psychometric properties of the QUALID and CILQ scales. *Aging & Mental Health.* 2017, 21:1287-1293. IF 2.663.

Bužgová, R., Bar, M...Kozáková, R., Zeleníková, R., et al. Neuropalliative and rehabilitative care in patients with an advanced stage of progressive neurological diseases. *Česká a slovenská neurologie a neurochirurgie.* 2018, 81(1): 17-23. IF 0.508.

Bužgová, R., Janíková, E. Czech adaption of the Collet-Lester fear of death scale in a sample of nursing students. *OMEGA-Journal of death and dying.* 2017 first online. doi.org/10.1177/0030222817725183. IF 0.870.

Bužgová, R., Kozáková, R. Psychometric evaluation of a Czech version of the Family Inventory of Needs. *Palliative and Supportive Care.* 2016, 14(2):142-150. IF 1.211.

Bužgová, R., Kozáková, R., Juríčková L. The unmet needs of patients with progressive neurological diseases in the Czech republic: a qualitative study. *Journal of Palliative Care.* 2019, 34(1): 38-46. IF 0.882.

Bužgová, R., Sikorova, L., Jarošová, D. Assessing Patients' Palliative Care Needs in the Final Stages of Illness During Hospitalization. *American Journal of Hospice and Palliative Medicine.* 2016, 33(2): 184-193. IF 1.347.

Bužgová, R., Sikorová, L., KozákovÁ R., et al. Predictors of change in quality of life in patients with end-stage disease during hospitalization. *Journal of palliative care.* 2017, 32(2):69-76. IF 0.882.

Bužgová, R., Špatenková, N. Assessing needs of family members of inpatients with advanced cancer. *European Journal of Cancer Care.* 2016, 25:592-599. IF 1.564.

Charalambous, A.,... Bužgová R. The quality of oncology nursing care: a cross sectional survey in three countries in Europe. *European Journal of Oncology Nursing.* 2017, 27:45-52. IF 1.812.

Kozáková, R., Bužgová, R., Zeleníková, R. Mobbing of nurses: prevalence, forms and psychological consequences in the Moravian-silesian region. *Československá psychologie.* 2018, 62(4): 316-329. IF 0.193.

Siverová, J., Bužgová, R. The effect of reminiscence therapy on quality of life, attitudes to ageing, and depressive symptoms in institutionalized elderly adults with cognitive impairment: A quasi-experimental study. *International journal of mental health nursing.* 2018, 27(5):1430-1439. IF 2.033.

INDEX

A

adenosine, 28
adenosine triphosphate, 28
aluminum, v, vii, viii, 27, 28, 30, 31, 51, 54, 55, 56, 57, 58, 59, 60, 61, 62, 63, 64, 65, 70, 71
aluminum neurotoxicity, v, viii, 27, 28, 51, 54, 57, 61, 62, 63, 64
amino, 29, 34, 38, 46, 50, 67
amino acid, 29, 34, 38, 46, 50, 67
Amyotrophic Lateral Sclerosis, 37, 48, 49, 66, 67, 68, 89, 91, 93
aspartate, 29

B

beta-lactam antibiotics, 29, 30, 40, 43, 53, 64, 65

C

calcium homeostasis, 33, 51, 69
ceftriaxone, v, vii, viii, 27, 28, 30, 31, 40, 43, 44, 45, 46, 47, 48, 49, 50, 51, 52, 54, 55, 58, 59, 60, 61, 62, 63, 64, 67, 68, 69, 70
convulsion(s), 52, 53, 70
cytochrome c oxydase, 58

D

disorder(s), vii, viii, ix, 2, 4, 5, 7, 8, 9, 10, 12, 16, 19, 22, 23, 24, 25, 28, 30, 33, 37, 44, 47, 48, 50, 51, 67, 71, 75, 86, 88
dying, 74, 94, 95

E

Epilepsy, 17, 37, 52, 53, 54, 69
excitatory amino acid transporter, 29, 34, 38, 46, 50, 67
experimental design, 54

F

free radicals, 33, 57, 59, 60, 62

G

GABA, 37, 38
glucose, ix, 28, 56, 57, 58, 71
glucose-6-phosphate dehydrogenase, ix, 28, 56, 57, 58, 71
glutamate, 29, 39, 66
glutamate (GABA)-glutamine cycle, 37, 38
glutamate excitotoxicity, 29, 37, 47, 48, 50, 54, 62, 64
glutamate homeostasis, 31, 33, 35, 50
glutamate transporter 1, 29, 66
glutamate transporters, 31, 33, 34, 35, 36, 39, 40, 48, 52, 66, 69, 70
glutamate-aspartate transporter, 29
glutamate-mediated excitotoxicity, 39

H

health-care system, 75

I

immunoadsorption, 2, 6, 12, 15, 20, 21, 23, 24, 25
immunologic diseases, viii, 2
immunological disorders, 2

M

multidisciplinary team, 74, 82, 84, 85, 88

N

neurodegenerative diseases, viii, 28, 30, 40, 47, 52, 59, 62, 64
neurodegenerative disorders, 29, 47, 48, 93
neurologic diseases, 2, 7, 11
neurological diseases, 8, 18, 19, 44, 74, 79, 80, 87, 88, 89, 90, 91, 95
neurology, 22, 23, 74, 89, 90, 91, 92, 93
neuropalliative rehabilitation, ix, 74, 80, 88
neuroprotective potential, 46, 67
neurotoxicity, viii, 28, 30, 43, 45, 54, 61, 65, 68, 69, 71
nitrosative, 33

O

oxidative, viii, 28, 30, 33, 36, 46, 48, 51, 53, 54, 57, 58, 59, 60, 61, 62, 63, 64, 67, 68, 69
oxidative stress, viii, 28, 30, 36, 46, 48, 51, 53, 54, 57, 59, 60, 61, 62, 64, 67, 68, 69

P

palliative, ix, 73, 74, 75, 76, 78, 79, 80, 83, 84, 85, 86, 87, 88, 89, 90, 91, 92, 93, 94, 95
palliative care, ix, 73, 74, 75, 76, 78, 79, 80, 83, 84, 85, 86, 87, 88, 89, 90, 91, 92, 93, 94, 95
participants, ix, 49, 74, 76, 77, 78, 83
patients, v, vii, ix, 8, 9, 10, 13, 14, 15, 17, 18, 19, 20, 21, 23, 24, 30, 48, 49, 50, 51, 52, 53, 69, 73, 74, 75, 76, 77, 78, 80, 81, 82, 83, 84, 85, 86, 87, 88, 89, 90, 91, 92, 93, 95
pharmacotherapeutics, 39
phosphate, ix, 28, 56, 57, 58, 71
progressive, v, vii, ix, 8, 10, 11, 17, 18, 47, 48, 50, 73, 74, 76, 80, 83, 90, 92, 95

Q

qualitative research, ix, 73, 76, 78, 90, 91, 93
qualitative study, v, 73, 89, 90, 91, 95

quality of life, 52, 74, 75, 78, 80, 83, 87, 88, 90, 91, 93, 94, 95, 96

R

reduced glutathione, ix, 28, 56, 59, 60, 62
regulators, 39
rehabilitation, v, ix, 73, 74, 76, 77, 78, 80, 81, 82, 84, 86, 88, 94

S

screening, 39, 40
stress, ix, 28, 33, 46, 57, 59, 60
support, ix, 18, 19, 22, 74, 75, 76, 79, 80, 81, 82, 84, 85, 87, 88

supportive care, ix, 10, 30, 74, 80, 81, 87
synaptic cleft, 29, 32, 33, 35, 37

T

targets, 30, 39, 57, 64, 69
therapeutic apheresis, vii, 1, 2, 7, 17, 20, 21, 22, 23, 24
therapeutic plasma exchange, viii, 2, 21, 22, 23, 24, 25
transporters, 32, 33, 34, 35, 36, 37, 38, 40, 43, 68

U

unmet needs, 76, 90, 95

Related Nova Publications

A Closer Look at Motor-Evoked Potential

Editor: Shapour Jaberzadeh

Series: Neuroscience Research Progress

Book Description: This book is an update concerning the use of transcranial magnetic stimulation (TMS) as an assessment tool for the measurement of corticospinal excitability in interventional and non-interventional studies.

Hardcover ISBN: 978-1-53614-389-8
Retail Price: $160

Functional Neuroimaging Methods and Frontiers

Author: Yongxia Zhou, Ph.D.

Series: Neuroscience Research Progress

Book Description: The aim of this book is intended to provide a whole picture of new fMRI imaging methodological developments from principles to applications, to both beginners and experts in biomedical imaging and healthcare.

Softcover ISBN: 978-1-53614-123-8
Retail Price: $95

To see a complete list of Nova publications, please visit our website at www.novapublishers.com

Related Nova Publications

ARTIFICIAL INTELLIGENCE DRIVEN BY A GENERAL NEURAL SIMULATION SYSTEM (GENESIS)

AUTHORS: Bahman Zohuri and Masoud Moghaddam

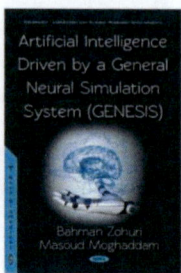

SERIES: Neurology – Laboratory and Clinical Research Developments

BOOK DESCRIPTION: The last several years have seen a dramatic increase in the number of neurobiologists building or using computer-based models as a regular part of their efforts to understand how different neural systems function.

HARDCOVER ISBN: 978-1-53613-196-3
RETAIL PRICE: $310

MOVEMENT 2018: BRAIN, BODY AND COGNITION

AUTHORS: Joav Merrick, MD, MMedSci, DMSc and Gerry Leisman, MD, PhD

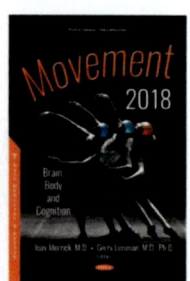

SERIES: Functional Neurology

BOOK DESCRIPTION: This book is based on the conference on "Movement and Cognition" held in July 2018 at the Joseph B. Martin Center at Harvard Medical School in Boston, where an opportunity was provided for researchers and practitioners from various disciplines to share their knowledge and experience in an academic environment that has supported learning and social change for hundreds of years.

HARDCOVER ISBN: 978-1-53614-833-6
RETAIL PRICE: $310

To see a complete list of Nova publications, please visit our website at www.novapublishers.com